HIPAA for Medical Office Personnel

DAN KRAGER

CAROLE KRAGER

THOMSON

DELMAR LEARNING

Australia   Canada   Mexico   Singapore   Spain   United Kingdom   United States

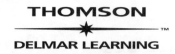

THOMSON

DELMAR LEARNING

HIPAA for Medical Office Personnel
by Dan Krager and Carole Krager

Vice President, Health Care Business Unit:
William Brottmiller

Editorial Director:
Cathy L. Esperti

Acquisitions Editor:
Rhonda Dearborn

Developmental Editor:
Sarah Duncan

Marketing Director:
Jennifer McAvey

Marketing Coordinator:
Kimberly Duffy

Editorial Assistant:
Debra Gorgos

Production Editor:
Anne Sherman

Library of Congress Cataloging-in-Publication Data

Krager, Dan.
  HIPAA for medical office personnel / Dan Krager and Carole Krager.
    p. ; cm.
  Includes bibliographical references and index.
  ISBN 1-4018-6574-7 (alk. paper)
    1. United States. Health Insurance Portability and Accountability Act of 1996. 2. Insurance, Health—Continuation coverage—Law and legislation—United States.
3. Medical assistants—United States—Handbooks, manuals, etc.
I. Title: Health Insurance Portability and Accountability Act for medical office personnel. II. Krager, Carole.
III. Title.
    KF3515.3.K73 2005
    344.7302'2—dc22
                            2004013510

NOTICE TO THE READER

Contents

Introduction   vii
About the Authors   ix
Acknowledgments   xi

Chapter 1 Introduction to HIPAA   **1**
Chapter Outline   1
Key Terms   2
Think About It   2
True Stories   2
    Introduction   4
    Overview of the Rulings   5
    Development of the Rulings   5
    Titles in HIPAA   6
        Title I: Health Insurance Access, Portability, and Renewal   6
        Title II: Preventing Health Care Fraud and Abuse   6
        Title III: Tax-related Provisions   7
        Title IV: Group Health Plan Requirements   7
        Title V: Revenue Offsets   7
        Other Titles in HIPAA   7
            Title XI: General Provisions, Peer Review, and Administrative
                Simplification   7
            Title XXVII: Assuring Portability, Availability and Renewability of
                Health Insurance Coverage   8
    HIPAA: An Organizational and Business Challenge   8
Summary   11
End of Chapter Questions   12
Scenarios   12
References   13

39.95

8-29-07

Chapter 2 Privacy Issues Explained   15

Chapter Outline   15
Key Terms   16
Think About It   16
True Stories   16
Introduction   17
  To Whom Does Title II Apply?   17
  Who is a "Covered Entity"?   18
  The HIPAA Officer   19
  Locating the Latest Title II Rules and Changes   20
  What is Protected Health Information?   21
    Authorization Versus Consent   22
    Protected Health Information Concerns and Disclosures 23
    Required Disclosures   24
    Permitted Use and Disclosure Without Authorization 24
      For Individual Access   24
      For Treatment, Payment, and Health Care Operations 24
      When Permission to Disclose is Obtained 24
      Disclosures that are Incidental   25
      Disclosures for Public Interest or to Benefit the Public 26
      Disclosures for Research   27
    Permitted Use and Disclosure With Authorization   27
      Disclosure of Psychotherapy Notes 27
      Disclosure for Marketing Purposes 27
    Limiting Uses and Disclosures   28
    Minimum Necessary Uses   28
  Business Associates under Privacy Ruling   29
  Training of Workforce and the Public   29
  Enforcement Guidelines   30
Summary   31
End of Chapter Questions   32
Scenarios   33
References   34

Chapter 3 Transaction Standards and Code Sets   35

Chapter Outline   35
Key Terms   36
Think About It   36
Introduction   36
  Purpose of Transaction Standards   37
  Designated Code Sets   39
    Diagnosis Codes   39
    Inpatient Procedure Codes   40
    Outpatient Procedure Codes   40
    Dental Procedure Codes   41
    Drug Codes   41

Non-medical Code Sets   42
ASC X12 Nomenclature   42
Data Overview   43
Architecture   43
Use of Loops   46
Sample of EDI Claim Data   48
Limitations to Claims Encounters   51
Remittance Advice and Secondary Payer   51
Working with Outside Entities   52
Trading Partner Agreements   52
Business Use and Definition   52
Summary   53
End of Chapter Questions   53
Scenarios   56
References   56

Chapter 4 HIPAA Security Ruling   57

Chapter Outline   57
Key Terms   58
Think About It   58
True Stories   58
Introduction   59
Core Requirements   59
Administrative Safeguards   61
Security Management   61
Assigned Security Responsibility—Security Officer   62
Workforce Security   63
Information Access   63
Security Awareness and Training   63
Security Incidents   64
Contingency Plan   64
Evaluation of Security Effectiveness   65
Business Associate Contracts   65
Physical Safeguards   65
Facility Access Controls   65
Workstation Use or Access   66
Workstation Security   66
Device and Media Controls   67
Technical Safeguards   67
Access Control   68
Audit Controls   69
Integrity   69
Person or Entity Authentication   69
Transmission Security   70
Organizational Requirements   70
Policies, Procedures, and Documentation   70

Impact on Organizations 71
Challenges to Compliance 72
Summary 73
End of Chapter Questions 74
Scenarios 75
References 84

Chapter 5 Unique Health Identifiers and Misconceptions **87**
Chapter Outline 87
Key Terms 88
Think About It 88
Introduction 88
  Reasons for Identification Numbers 88
    Employer Identifier 89
    Health Care Provider Identifier 90
    Health Plan Identifier 91
    Personal Identifier 91
  What is Important to Know About HIPAA? 94
  Misconceptions About HIPAA 94
Summary 98
End of Chapter Questions 99
Scenarios 100
References 100

Appendix A Resources for Further Information **99**

Appendix B Required and Addressable Security Standards **103**

Appendix C Further Scenarios and Questions for Consideration **107**

Glossary 109
Index 115

Introduction

This textbook is written specifically for the student taking courses in health care. This textbook will be useful for students studying medical office procedures or nursing, as certified nursing assistants, and in other medical fields. This text may also be useful for training new hospital personnel including housekeepers, physicians, clinic and physician employees, administrators, office managers, laboratory technicians, and health care clearinghouse workers. Each chapter has Think About It questions at the beginning of the chapter to stimulate reflection and Review Questions at the conclusion to solidify important points.

Since 1996 when Congress passed the Health Insurance Portability and Accountability Act, or HIPAA, the Department of Health and Human Services (DHHS) formulated federal rules for all health care providers, health plans, and health care clearinghouses. Compliance with these regulations is mandatory; ignorance of the rulings is not acceptable. Everyone whose work involves any health information must be knowledgable about the ruling so they can effectively provide care and services for patients. We have presented the rulings as proposed by the DHHS. Changes will take place as the rulings develop. Each provider is responsible to train all employees to understand compliance with the rulings. This textbook will give any student or employee a basic understanding of what the rulings are and how they affect each area of health care.

APPROACH TO THE TEXT

This textbook fills a need to address the HIPAA rulings mandated by the federal government that directly affect the delivery of health care. This book provides an overview of all sections of the HIPAA ruling. Specific chapters focus on matters of *privacy, electronic transmissions* of health information, *security* of health information, and *unique identifiers* to be used in the transmissions. Many other textbooks focus only on either Privacy Rules or Security Rules to the exclusion of the other.

The sources for this textbook are governmental rulings and government websites. A general understanding of the health care process is helpful for the best understanding of the text but those without health care experience will still gain an understanding of HIPAA rules.

ORGANIZATION

The text is divided into five chapters. Chapter 1 provides an overview of the complete federal ruling. The next chapters examine the four areas specified by Congress that impact the medical office and the health care provider. Chapter 2 explores what *privacy of protected health information* means. Chapter 3 explains *electronic transmissions of health information* and what mandated *code sets* to use in order to process health claims. Chapter 4 covers the *security measures* that must be in place to protect health information from an outside threat or a natural disaster. Included in Chapter 4 is a *scenario* of a typical hospital emergency encounter with follow-up stay showing where HIPAA rules intersect the health care services. Chapter 5 has two parts: explanation of various *identifiers* to be included in the transactions and also explanations of some *myths about what HIPAA does or does not mean.* Appendix A lists many websites for further exploration of HIPAA regulations directly from government sources. Appendix B charts the Security Rule and whether rulings are required or addressable. Appendix C contains an expanded list of questions and situations to help the student understand how HIPAA rulings are interpreted in day-to-day experiences.

FEATURES

Each chapter has *Think About It* questions to stimulate reflection about the subject of the chapter. These questions are included to encourage debate. The end of each chapter includes a summary and review questions that reinforce learning of important concepts. True stories are included in the text that point out the need for HIPAA regulations. Scenarios illustrate how these rulings relate to real life situations. In order to better understand electronic transactions a detailed example is given showing information printed on a paper claim and then as a data string. Another feature is a step-by-step sequence of an individual entering a hospital for health care, and an explanation of how HIPAA privacy, security, and electronic transaction rules are applicable.

SUPPLEMENTAL MATERIALS FOR THE TEACHER

The teaching package for the instructor includes:
   —Topics for discussion from *Think About It* questions
   —Answers to the review questions at the end of each chapter
   —An outline of how the chapters can be incorporated into a text that covers instruction
      for people working in the medical office setting

About the Authors

Carole Krager has 20 years' experience teaching in public schools and four years' experience in the community college setting. She has firsthand experience with hospital-based clinic billing of insurance claims, claims adjustments, and submitting claims electronically for faster reimbursement. Trained through Triton College in diagnostic coding, Carole has experience in outpatient coding for a 104-bed hospital with lab, radiology, physical, respiratory, and occupational therapy departments. She has taught medical insurance and coding at Olney Central College, part of Illinois Eastern Community College in Olney, Illinois. She is a member of AHIMA, the American Health Information Management Association.

Dan Krager has over 15 years' experience in computer software and hardware applications. He has managed computer systems in three hospitals, bringing many innovations that allow health care data to be electronically and securely transmitted. He is currently HIPAA Officer and Security Officer for the 108-bed Richland Memorial Hospital in Olney, Illinois. He is responsible for HIPAA training for all personnel and HIPAA compliance issues dealing with electronic transmissions and security. He has delegated Privacy Officer duties to a Risk Manager.

Acknowledgments

We wish to acknowledge some persons who have greater expertise in specific areas than we have. Their contributions and suggestions helped to assure that information is accurate. They are: Deb Rann, Emergency Department Nurse, Lezlie Lambird, Director of Medical Records Department, and Ron Wallace, Director of Patient Financial Services. All work for Richland Memorial Hospital in Olney, Illinois. The drawings are by Nancy Hennessey of Olney, Illinois. Her sketches help express our concepts visually. We are very grateful for her enthusiastic contributions.

The authors and Publisher would like to thank the following reviewers for their feedback and suggestions at the manuscript stage:

Frank Harbison, B.S. Ed
Manager of Education
Vatterott College
Sunset Hills, Missouri

Fred Valdes, MD
Medical Department Chair
City College
Ft. Lauderdale, Forida

Lynn G. Slack, CMA
Medical Program Director
ICM School of Business & Medical Careers
Pittsburg, Pennsylvania

Lynette M. Veach, MA, MLT (ASCP)
Medical Assistant Instructor, retired
Aristotle Institute and Columbus State
    Community College
Columbus, Ohio

AVENUE FOR FEEDBACK

Contact may be made through email: dkrager@otbnet.com

1

Introduction to HIPAA

CHAPTER OUTLINE

Introduction

Overview of the Rulings

Development of the Rulings

Titles in HIPAA

Title I: Health Insurance Access, Portability, and Renewal

Title II: Preventing Health Care Fraud and Abuse

Title III: Tax-related Provisions

Title IV: Group Health Plan Requirements

Title V: Revenue Offsets

Other Titles in HIPAA

Title XI: General Provisions, Peer Review, and Administrative Simplification

Title XXVII: Assuring Portability, Availability, and Renewability of Health Insurance Coverage

HIPAA: An Organizational and Business Challenge

Summary

KEY TERMS

group health plan

health care clearinghouse

health care provider

Health Insurance Portability and
Accountability Act of 1996 (HIPAA)

Medical Savings Account (MSA)

privacy

transaction

THINK ABOUT IT

1. Give an example of what you have heard about the ruling called HIPAA.

2. Why does the HIPAA ruling stir up so much talk?

3. Debate the reasons for keeping health information private. What are reasons for disclosure? What are reasons for privacy?

4. Give examples of how people might be hurt when certain medical information is revealed to: employers, family members, social friends, and financial organizations.

True Story

An Atlanta truck driver lost his job in early 1998 after his employer learned from his insurance company that he had sought treatment for a drinking problem.

—Appleby, 2000

True Story

Thousands of medical records fell out of a vehicle and were blown throughout Mesa, Arizona. The records were being transported to be destroyed.

—Medical Records Fall Out, 2000

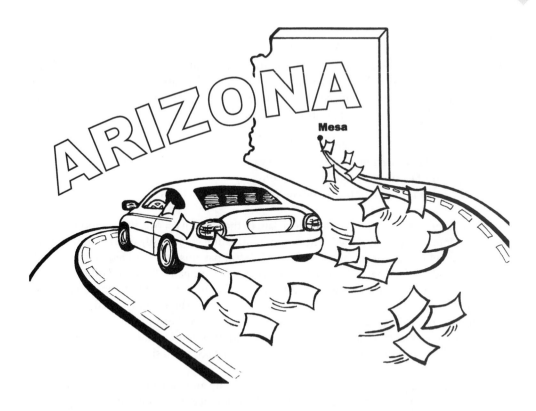

True Story

After suffering a work-related injury to her wrist, Roni Breite authorized her insurance company to release information pertaining to her wrist ailment to her employer. When she had the opportunity to review her medical records, the file contained her entire medical history, including records on recent fertility treatment and pregnancy loss.

—McCarthy, 1999

True Story

In Maryland, eight Medicaid clerks were prosecuted for selling computerized record print-outs of recipients' and dependents' financial resources to sales representatives of managed care companies.

—Forbes, 1996

INTRODUCTION

The **Health Insurance Portability and Accountability Act of 1996**, now known as HIPAA, mandates many changes to health insurance carriers and health care providers. There are four main areas where the law has changed the way business is conducted for those in the health care industry. We will cover each of these areas in chapter discussions.

1. *Privacy* of health information
2. Standards for *electronic transactions* of health information and claims
3. *Security* of electronic health information
4. *National identifiers* for the parties in health care transactions

First look at the general picture of the federal law. In the accounts above, information that was not public information was shared. The health information could easily be used to restrict or terminate employment, or in the case of the Medicaid patients and families, be used to sell insurance products for financial gain of the managed care company. These and other accounts began to accumulate and pressure was subsequently placed on Congress to enact legislation that would safeguard anyone's medical information no matter where they traveled in the country. Since the mid 1970s, U.S. representatives and senators have been proposing legislation to reform various elements of the health care industry. Most proposals failed and a compromise was not reached until 1996, when the 104th Congress focused upon six issues:

1. To improve portability and continuity in the group and individual insurance markets
2. To combat waste, fraud, and abuse in health insurance and health care delivery
3. To promote the use of Medical Savings Accounts (MSA)
4. To improve access to long-term care services and coverage
5. To simplify the administration of health insurance
6. To provide a means to pay for reforms, and other related purposes

Representative Bill Archer of Texas, along with 25 other sponsors, presented House Bill #3103 to amend the Internal Revenue Code of 1986. The Health Insurance Portability and Accountability Act of 1996 passed both houses of Congress and became Public Law 104-191. Congress included many related issues within the seven titles of the bill. By signing this bill President Clinton confirmed a process that generated new rules for health insurance plans and health care providers in addition to penalties for non-compliance. The law is subdivided into seven titles:

Title I—Health Care Access, Portability, and Renewability
Title II—Preventing Health Care Fraud and Abuse; Administrative Simplification; Medical Liability Reform
Title III—Tax-related Health Provisions
Title IV—Application and Enforcement of Group Health Plan Requirements
Title V—Revenue Offsets
Title XI—General Provisions, Peer Review, Administrative Simplification
Title XXVII—Assuring Portability, Availability, and Renewability of Health Insurance Coverage
    H.R. 3103 (1996).

The reason the titles are not sequential is that not all portions (titles) of the original bill passed the compromise legislation. Legislative business demands that compromises be made to develop agreements. The ruling addresses real concerns in the health insurance industry. With health insurance changes came other adjustments leading to ways in which health information is handled. The inclusion of Title II—Administrative Simplification affects practices and procedures of **health care providers**. A health care provider is anyone or organization who furnishes, bills, or is paid for health care in the normal course of business.

There were many unfinished details that Congress did not address when they adopted this law. They included a provision in the law that if the details were not addressed in a timely manner (within three years of passage of HIPAA), the task of addressing the details would fall to the Department of Health and Human Services (DHHS). Congress left the details to the secretary of the DHHS to develop rulings in accordance with Public Law 104-191 or HIPAA. Since the DHHS rulings are not law, the DHHS can adjust, amend, delete, or change the rulings at any time. Modifications to the first rulings are already being issued.

OVERVIEW OF THE RULINGS

In October 1997, Representative David Hobson presented a clarification of HIPAA. In short, he referred to the fact that "a few people do not want to play by the rules." Since this is often true, Congress has written law that mandates standards for all payers of health care. This simplifies the administration of medical billing procedures because industry-wide standards will be used to electronically transmit all transactions by means of electronic data interchange (EDI). "Providers are given the option of whether to conduct the transactions electronically or 'on paper' but if they elect to conduct them electronically, they must use the standards agreed upon through the law" (Hobson, 1997). Payers are required to accept these transmissions and are not to delay a transaction or adversely affect the provider who conducts transactions electronically. Representative Hobson's intent is that all covered entities will be treated equally regarding payment from payers for health care. Failure for noncompliance is clearly outlined. The goal is to "simplify the administration of the nation's health care system and improve its efficiency and effectiveness" (Hobson, 1997). The DHHS wrote rulings so that all parties large and small would have to comply. With a nation-wide standard, all entities in the health insurance process will be able to interact with greater ease. Small private insurance providers and government agencies will be treated equally and they must treat each health care provider the same. The flow of information and reimbursements will become faster and more efficient. This will result in savings in the cost of insurance and providing health care. By studying the concepts presented here, you will be confident that you can work in the health care industry without fear of the HIPAA rules.

DEVELOPMENT OF THE RULINGS

In 1998, the DHHS began developing details of the rules. They proposed rulings and published them for review. Anyone can then submit comments to the DHHS about the rulings and suggest changes. After an extensive period of comment and public hearings, an implementation team reviews and analyzes the comments. The implementation team is responsible for the final content of the ruling. Then the secretary of the DHHS approves the final rules. The secretary releases the rules in the Federal Register and to the public. An effective date is determined for enforcement. Compliance by all parties is required 24 months after the effective date. Once a ruling is adopted it will be in force for a period of at least 12 months. All parties affected by HIPAA are required to keep up to date with any changes. The responsibility lies with each organization under HIPAA rules. Health care providers will need to continue to refer to the current directives of the DHHS to see how the rules change over time.

TITLES IN HIPAA

Following are all titles covered by the entire HIPAA law. The focus is on providing a means for people to carry insurance coverage from one health insurance company to another and to simplify communication between health insurance plans and health care providers. We provide a short overview of each portion.

Title I: Health Insurance Access, Portability, and Renewal

Title I (1): Health Care Access Portability and Renewability amends the Employee Retirement Income Security Act of 1974 (ERISA) and the Public Health Act by increasing the portability of health insurance. It changes the rules concerning preexisting condition exclusions. When a worker changes jobs or is released from work, he can continue health coverage even with a preexisting condition. This ruling prohibits discrimination based on health status in regard to health insurance coverage. It also guarantees renewability for certain group health plans.

Title II: Preventing Health Care Fraud and Abuse

Title II (2): Preventing Health Care Fraud and Abuse; Administrative Simplification; Medical Liability Reform is the portion of the bill that speaks to health providers and how they interact with the insurance network.

The important areas of concern seek to:

1. prevent fraud and abuse in the delivery of and payment for health care.
2. improve the Medicare program and other programs through efficient and effective standards.
3. establish standards and requirements for all electronic transmission of certain health information. H.R. 3103 (1996).

Title II establishes a fraud and abuse control program as well as a means of collecting health information. It spells out civil and criminal penalties for guilty parties when either abuse or fraud events are documented. Each state has enacted regulations governing the health insurance companies within their jurisdiction. Each state has regulations concerning abuse. Only federal programs, such as Medicare, Medicaid, TRICARE, and CHAMPVA, have federal authority to prosecute situations of fraud. With the HIPAA ruling governing transactions in all 50 states, some state rules will be preempted by the jurisdiction of the federal ruling. All covered entities are obligated to comply with the federal law as a minimum no matter where they are located. Only when state or local laws are more stringent will the state or local law be held as the standard for the providers in that particular area.

Title III: Tax-related Provisions

Title III (3): Tax-related Health Provisions addresses Medical Savings Accounts (MSA) and how employers handle these funds for employees, increasing the deduction for health insurance for self-employed individuals, long-term care insurance benefits, related consumer protection provisions, and income tax refund payments in relation to organ and tissue donations. A **Medical Savings Account (MSA)** is a tax-sheltered savings account similar to an Individual Retirement Account (IRA), but earmarked for medical expenses only. Participating individuals can deposit money into this type of account and withdraw the funds throughout the year for medical expenses only. Deposits are 100% tax-deductible for the self-employed and can be withdrawn by check or debit card to pay routine medical bills with tax-free dollars.

Title IV: Group Health Plan Requirements

Title IV (4): Application and Enforcement of Group Health Plan Requirements amends the Consolidated Omnibus Budget Reconciliation Act of 1985 (COBRA). It details how group health plans must allow for portability, access, and renewability for members of a group health plan. A **group health plan** is defined as an employee welfare benefit plan that provides health coverage in the form of medical care and services through insurance, reimbursement, or other means for a group of employees and dependents. It may be sponsored by an employer or a labor union and includes private employer plans, federal governmental plans, non-federal governmental plans, and church plans. Many employers have arrangements for employees to participate in a health plan that includes any person employed by the organization—thus the group health plan. As workers move from one job to another, this ruling allows people the option of carrying the same health insurance coverage to their new work situation, instead of having to start over again with waiting periods for preexisting conditions or other similar conditions of coverage.

Title V: Revenue Offsets

Title V (5): Revenue Offsets explains how the ruling changed the Internal Revenue Code of 1986 to generate more revenue to offset the HIPAA required costs.

Other Titles in HIPAA

The other two titles in the bill cover minor issues and are short in length. They clarify certain items of the law.

Title XI: General Provisions. Title XI (11): General Provisions, Peer Review, and Administrative Simplification explains that these provisions are to be coordinated with Medicare-related plans and are not a duplication of coverage.

Title XXVII: Assuring Portability. Title XXVII (27): Assuring Portability, Availability, and Renewability of Health Insurance Coverage is written specifically for health insurance plans to ensure that employee coverage will be carried over from one plan to another.

HIPAA: An Organizational and Business Challenge

Health insurance plans, **health care clearinghouses**, payers of medical insurance, and other associated businesses have to adjust their practices to be in compliance with these titles. A health care clearinghouse is a business that submits health claims on behalf of a provider. Their function is to screen the claim for accuracy and be the intermediary between the health care provider and the insurance carrier. The Administrative Simplification portion of HIPAA has caused many changes within physician offices, clinics, hospitals, and outpatient offices.

In 2003, the Centers for Medicare and Medicaid Services (CMS) verified that there are over 400 different ways to submit a health insurance claim. This means delays in payment and too much time spent by the medical billing assistant customizing each claim to the specifications of a particular insurance carrier. Only a federal law could compel all 50 states to comply with one standard. Many health insurance companies have headquarters that serve several states. Each state may have standards unique to itself. Health insurance carriers can also demand certain forms and/or styles of claims submission. The Blue Cross and Blue Shield plans, for instance, have a unique requirement to designate units of service on the current outpatient claim form. A number of health insurance companies request a separate form along with the claim in order to process claims. This federal ruling requires one standard form for submission of health claims. The HIPAA ruling will also eliminate having to customize claims before they are submitted for payment. The title of "Administrative Simplification" describes the hope of this ruling. Business office personnel can submit one form electronically, with confidence that as long as codes and patient data information are accurate, the claim will be paid in a timely manner. Gone are the various forms used by companies and their unique requirements. Fewer claims will be rejected because information was not accepted as submitted. The government has ruled the claims submission process be standardized to a single format for all parties. Providers will be paid faster and benefits between health plans will be coordinated quickly.

Health care providers are not required by HIPAA to conduct any transactions electronically, although Medicare is definitely moving in that direction at this time. However, if health care providers transmit even one claim electronically, they will need to comply with the HIPAA standardized electronic format. Private insurance companies are also pushed in this direction because the electronic process has the potential for significant savings. Greater efficiency will be a result of this change. The supply of paper, the sorting of paper, the storage and final long-term archival storage of paper is currently a large cost of doing business. A study has shown that it takes at least seven people to manage

Seven people manage one piece of paper.

Someone fills it with data.

Someone authenticates it.

Someone has to distribute it.

Someone converts the data to meaningful information (reads it or makes a report).

Someone has to file it.

Someone has to retrieve it.

Someone has to manage the final disposition of it whether stored or destroyed.

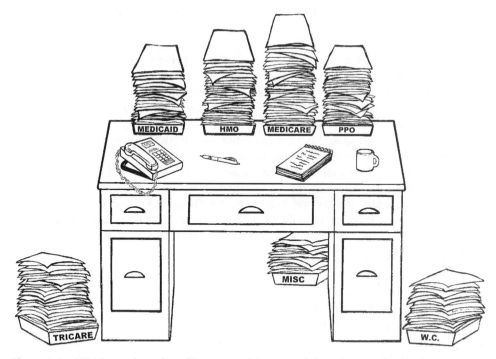

Figure 1-1   HIPAA mandates that all insurance claims must follow the same format, thus simplifying administrative paperwork.

one single piece of paper. Few providers have even considered a disaster plan to protect or replace lost paper records. With electronic data and transmissions, the need for paper, the accompanying file cabinets, and the space to house the cabinets will be a thing of the past.

First the rule for Unique Health Identifiers for Employers was presented and finalized. The deadline for compliance was July 30, 2002. This ruling stipulates that employers must use a unique identification number on any electronic transmission. This number has been designated as the Employer Identification Number (EIN) issued by the Internal Revenue Service for tax purposes. This portion of HIPAA was adopted without much disruption in the health industry. Other identifiers are to be standardized: physicians, health plans, and possibly personal/patient identifiers. Since this ruling is not complete, we will address this codification of identification in the last chapter.

The second portion finalized was the Privacy Rule from Title II Administrative Simplification, and the deadline for compliance was established as April 14, 2003. The Privacy Rule addressed the following three issues:

1. The rights that an individual should have who is a subject of *individually identifiable health information* (IIHI).
2. The procedures that should be established for the exercise of such rights.

3. The uses and disclosures of such information that should be authorized or required. H.R. 3101 (1996).

This ruling caused many false rumors about the meaning of **privacy** and how it would play out in the life of the medical community. The most general definition of privacy is an individual's claim to control the use and disclosure of personal information. HIPAA seeks to ensure that an individual's health information is kept confidential. The law outlines how health information may be shared or disclosed so that medical treatment is not hindered.

The Transaction and Code Set Rule mandates industry-wide standards for electronic transmission of protected health information. The Transaction and Code Set Rule deadline was set at October 16, 2003. The DHHS authorized adoption of standards so electronic transmissions of insurance claims and other health information would use the same format for any health care insurance plan and any health care provider. The DHHS has adopted medical code sets currently in use by private and public parties for medical concepts and also adopted other codes to efficiently transmit data. The transactions referred to are those that include:

- ❖ Health insurance claims
- ❖ Enrollment and ending enrollment in a health plan
- ❖ Eligibility for a health plan
- ❖ Health care payment and remittance advice
- ❖ Health plan premium payments
- ❖ First report of injury for workers' compensation claims
- ❖ Referral certification and authorization

By standardizing these transactions, the administration of health claims will be simplified from what was required prior to the ruling. Health claims can be filed electronically, edited by computer software for errors, and those that are deemed accurate can be paid electronically. The health care provider receives payment almost immediately by an electronic transfer of funds to the provider's bank account. Paper claims usually take four to six weeks to be returned with payment. The cash flow for the medical office is greatly accelerated. Claims submitted with errors take more time to correct and be processed.

The Security Rule requires safeguards to ensure the integrity of the protected health information. Because any electronically submitted health information is regulated, each office must have certain pieces of hardware and software in place to comply with HIPAA. As an employee, one should be aware of these rules without necessarily having to be directly responsible for the technical aspects. Care should be given to follow all guidelines for transmission, storage, and protection of all data and information. The Security Rule deadline was established as April 21, 2005. Security standards take into account:

- ❖ The technical capabilities of record systems used to maintain health information
- ❖ The costs of security measures
- ❖ The need for training persons who have access to health information
- ❖ The value of audit trails in computerized record systems
- ❖ The needs and capabilities of small health care providers and rural health care providers

Because health information is increasingly sent via electronic media, there is a real need to ensure that this information is kept secure while being transmitted. Just as some people can decode cell phone numbers, medical information can be illegally retrieved while it is being sent via a communication system. Security of electronic health information is of utmost priority. Certain procedures need to be in place to assure confidentiality and protect against loss. The Security Rule addresses these issues.

Some deadlines have been extended one year to accommodate the limited resources of small health care providers to comply. A small provider or supplier is a physician, practitioner, facility, or a supplier with fewer than 10 full-time employees. Another category of small providers is defined as hospitals, critical access hospitals, skilled nursing facilities, comprehensive outpatient rehabilitation facilities, home health agencies, or hospice programs with fewer than 25 full-time employees. These organizations generally have another 12 months to be in compliance.

SUMMARY

In 1996 Congress passed HIPAA. This law began a series of events reforming how health care insurance was managed by the insurance industry. The law provided rulings written by the DHHS standardizing the electronic processing of claims. These rulings simplified how health insurance claims are prepared and sent for payment. Insurance companies must provide individuals greater access to health care insurance when they change employers. They must also extend the coverage individuals need to new insurance carriers. Another insurance issue addressed is the use of MSA, which allows employees to set aside a certain amount of money to be used solely for health care in a year's time. Also written into the law are several ways to pay for these reforms.

Four important issues were addressed that change the way health care providers interact with their patients and insurance carriers. The first ruling established the Standard Unique Employer Identifier. By using the Internal Revenue Service's EIN employers can be uniquely identified in electronic transactions. Identifier standards are to be issued for health care providers, health plans, and patients. The next change was to provide all patients with a statement of how their protected health information is handled. The Privacy Ruling includes what information can be shared and also regulates how much and who can receive this information. The Privacy Ruling mandated that all patients must receive an explanation of how to protect their health information and lists safeguards that must be in place with each health care provider. The third change implemented is how the health care claim is processed. This mandated a uniform manner to electronically send and receive health care insurance claims. The Transaction Standards and Code Set Ruling standardizes all electronic claim formats and eliminates the many forms that insurance payers have insisted upon in the past. When protected health information is communicated through electronic means there is a need for security measures to be in place to protect it from loss or disclosure. The Security Ruling states how this is to be accomplished. Both the Transaction and Code Set Ruling and the Security Ruling involve information technology expertise.

Congress stressed that the goal of HIPAA is to simplify the insurance claim process and provide faster payments for services rendered by the health care provider. However, while these changes are being implemented many questions arise. Using explanations of this ruling and interpretations of the changes, one can understand the flow of protected health information through the medical office and the measures mandated to protect it from unauthorized disclosures.

END OF CHAPTER QUESTIONS

1. What are the four areas in which the DHHS mandated changes in the protection of health information?

2. What issues forced Congress to pass the HIPAA of 1996?

3. What government department issued the details of HIPAA?

4. If HIPAA and state laws are different, which takes precedence? Are there any exceptions?

5. Why is there a move to transmit medical insurance claims electronically? What advantages are there? What are the disadvantages?

6. Congress wrote an "Administrative Simplification" Title into the HIPAA bill. What is Congress hoping to simplify?

Scenarios

How would you answer?

Without knowing the details of the HIPAA rulings, how would you answer the following questions? As you study the following chapters, see if your first response was correct.

1. Many offices have sign-in sheets where patients are required to sign in as they enter. This gives the receptionist a priority list of who should be seen next. Is this list now banned from use? Why or why not? What are some other ways doctors' offices or clinics can get the same results?

2. A "Persons at Risk" program in New Jersey allows the Burlington Sheriff's Department to maintain a list of residents with severe mental health problems. The list is intended to help identify and locate people who may be lost or disoriented, but advocates are worried that the information could fall into the wrong hands or be used against people (New Jersey, 2000).

   a. If law enforcement officials do not know of these special residents, what negative results might occur?

   b. Do you consider this *an invasion of their privacy*?

3. Police in Fairfax, Virginia, seized records from a local drug treatment clinic when a car was stolen nearby. The police argued that the records were necessary to identify potential culprits, but returned the records after legal complaints were filed (Masters, 1998).

    a. If the records were inside the stolen car, was it wrong for the police to study them?

    b. How can patients at a drug treatment clinic keep their records protected?

4. Joan Kelly, an employee of Motorola, was automatically enrolled in a "depression program" by her employer after her prescription drugs management company reported that she was taking anti-depressants (O'Harrow, 1998).

    a. Is this an invasion of privacy?

    b. Should there be limits to the extent of health information an employer may have access to for any of his employees? Example: Should an employer find out how many employees have a diagnosis of hypertension?

5. In Maryland, eight Medicaid clerks were prosecuted for selling computerized records of recipients' and dependents' financial resources to sales representatives of managed care companies (*Forbes*, 1996).

    a. What part of HIPAA, if any, is aimed at preventing this?

REFERENCES

Appleby, J. (2002, March 23). File safe? Health records may not be confidential. *USA Today*, p. A1.

Forbes. (1996, May 20), p. 252.

Health Insurance Portability and Accountability Act of 1996, H.R. 3103, 104th Cong. (1996).

Hobson, Hon. David L. 105th Cong., E 2065. (1997, October 23).

Masters, B. (1998, September 1). Fairfax police concede seizure was wrong. *The Washington Post*, p. D1.

McCarthy, E. (1999, April 5). Patients voice growing concerns about privacy. *Sacramento Business Journal*.

Medical records fall out of vehicle, blown through streets. (2000, May 26). Associated Press.

New Jersey: Advocates angry over "Persons-at-Risk" list. (2000, May 30). *American HealthLine*.

O'Harrow, R. (1998, September 27). Plan's access to pharmacy data raises privacy issue. *The Washington Post*, p. A01.

Privacy Issues Explained

CHAPTER OUTLINE

Introduction

To Whom Does Title II Apply?

Who is a "Covered Entity"?

The HIPAA Officer

Locating the Latest Title II Rules and Changes

What is Protected Health Information?

Authorization Versus Consent

Protected Health Information Concerns and Disclosures

Required Disclosures

Permitted Use and Disclosure Without Authorization

For Individual Access

For Treatment, Payment, and Health Care Operations

When Permission to Disclose is Obtained

Disclosures that are Incidental

Disclosures for Public Interest or to Benefit the Public

Disclosures for Research

Permitted Use and Disclosure With Authorization

Disclosure of Psychotherapy Notes

Disclosure for Marketing Purposes

Limiting Uses and Disclosures

Minimum Necessary Uses

Business Associates under Privacy Ruling

Training of Workforce and the Public

Enforcement Guidelines

Summary

KEY TERMS

authorization

Business Associate (BA)

consent

covered entity

emancipated minor

de-identified health information

designated record set

disclosure (of protected health information)

health care operations

health plan

HIPAA Officer

incidental disclosure

individually identifiable health information (IIHI)

limited data set

marketing

minimum necessary

need to know

psychotherapy notes

protected health information (PHI)

treatment

use (of protected health information)

workforce

THINK ABOUT IT

1. Why might someone not want their medical records copied and sent to their employer?

2. What might be included in the records that would bias the employer against the worker?

3. What should you have received from a health provider about how it will handle your medical information after April 14, 2003?

True Story

A South Carolina resident was suspended from work for refusing to release her medical records to her employer.

—Crowley, 2000

True Story

The medical records of an Illinois woman were posted on the Internet without her knowledge or consent a few days after she was treated at St. Elizabeth's Medical Center following complications from an abortion at the Hope Clinic for Women. The woman has sued the hospital, alleging St. Elizabeth's released her medical records without her authorization to anti-abortion activists, who then posted the records online along with a photograph they had taken of her being transferred from the clinic to the hospital. The woman is also suing the anti-abortion activists for invading her privacy.

—Hillig and Mannies, 2001

INTRODUCTION

The privacy of personal information is an important issue for everyone. So much information is being shared today. Stores track purchases by individual identification, banks and other financial organizations submit information to credit organizations to provide credit ratings, closed-circuit cameras track many of our activities. With the move to protect our nation from outside terrorist activities, many enforcement agencies share information about individual activities. A federal rule about the use of personal health information must have safeguards to protect individuals from having private health information available to whomever may request it. The Department of Health and Human Services (DHHS) wrote the Privacy Rule to mandate nationwide standards to protect private health information.

TO WHOM DOES TITLE II APPLY?

The Health Insurance Portability and Accountability Act of 1996 (HIPAA), Public Law 104-191 was enacted on August 21, 1996. Sections 261 through 264 of the law required the secretary of the DHHS to publicize standards for the privacy of all health information. The goal of the ruling was to protect personal information while still allowing the flow of health information needed to properly and effectively treat patients to continue. The ruling was not intended to prevent health care givers from accessing information, or to cause delays that might bring harm to any patient through complicated steps of compliance. HIPAA clearly lists the circumstances when individual health information must be disclosed without an individual's authorization.

In April 2003, the first-ever federal privacy standards for medical data went into effect. Previously there were only state regulations concerning use and disclosure of medical records. There were many variations from state to state. Most doctors and medical offices realized that there needed to be limits on what information was released and to whom. Many people felt that their health information was open to anyone and everyone prior to April 2003. While this was not entirely true, as the vulnerability of electronic medical records became more widely known, people became very concerned. April 2003 was just the beginning of federal rulings to standardize how all patient information should be handled. With these rules a person could travel anywhere in the United States and expect the same safeguards to be in place.

Privacy issues are administrative in nature. Each health care provider must have certain policies in place to comply with the rulings. Many of these policies and practices will not be different from established medical office practices. Privacy compliance requires training staff to understand the rulings. Employees must follow certain policies for all the health care information they encounter in their work. Each office must make written policies available to all employees. If the Office of Civil Rights (OCR) conducts an investigation, the inspectors will expect to see written or electronic office policies and procedures. If policies are on paper *and* in electronic form, the inspectors will likely assume that the electronic system is not to be trusted. In such a case, they will expect to see the printed policy handbook. Although the guidelines seem strict, HIPAA allows for a great deal of flexibility. The Privacy Rule allows each organization to do "what is reasonable" within the guidelines. The rule does not specify how to comply. For example, to prevent conversations from being overheard does not mean that every time a physician speaks with a patient they must be in a room with the door closed. Reasonable and professional courtesy suggests that the physician ask visitors to leave the room or ask the patient if her care may be discussed with others present. As long as reasonable care is taken to comply with the intent of the ruling, and reasonable effort is documented, that will be sufficient.

WHO IS A "COVERED ENTITY"?

The term **covered entity** is part of the HIPAA language. There are three categories of covered entities. The first is any **health plan**. This is a company, individual, or group that agrees to pay part or all of the medical care for the people included in their coverage. There are many types of health plans—dental plans, vision plans, and prescription drug insurers in addition to the more traditional health insurance plans. Health plans include health maintenance organizations, Medicare, Medicaid, and Medicare+Choice. They also include Medicare supplemental insurers, Indian health service programs, veterans health care program (CHAMPVA), and Civilian Health and Medical Program of the Uniformed Services (CHAMPUS). Another type of entity that is covered is the long-term care insurer. An exception is given to an employer who has less than 50 employees and is "self-insured." (They pay for medical costs from their own funds within the company.) Only insurance companies who provide health coverage are included. These organizations are referred to as third-party payers. Insurance such as automobile, property, life, casualty, and workers' compensation are not health plans and do not come under this category.

The second type of covered entity is a *health care provider* who holds or transmits health information in any form or media whether electronic, paper, or oral. The privacy of personal health information is carefully outlined by the DHHS in the Privacy Rule. Any health information that is sent via electronic means must be kept secure from alteration, loss, and disclosure. The security measures are defined in the Security Rule. There are prior local laws and state statutes to protect health information that is in paper form. The Privacy Rule has defined protections for nationwide acceptance.

The third type of covered entity is a *health care clearinghouse*. This is a company that processes information it receives from health care providers and sends that information as an insurance claim for payment. In a small office a doctor may choose to send the billing task to

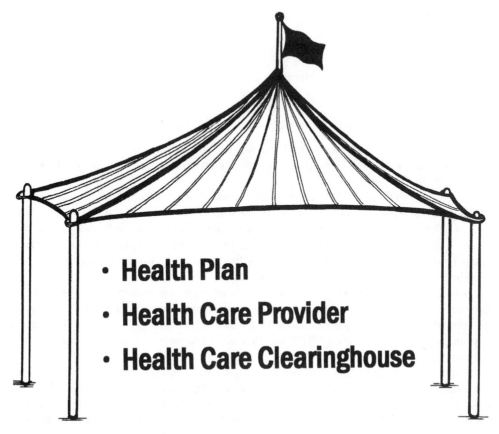

Figure 2-1 Only three types of organizations are required by the federal government to be in compliance with HIPAA regulations.

someone else whose business it is to keep abreast of changing rules. Clearinghouses handle claims from many providers and submit them in batches for processing. This allows the physician's office staff to concentrate on working with patients. The doctor pays a fee to the clearinghouse to send and receive insurance information for him. The clearinghouse will send the doctor credits from insurance payments minus their charge for the service. These clearinghouses are considered to be covered entities.

THE HIPAA OFFICER

One person in each covered entity is the designated **HIPAA Officer** who coordinates and oversees the various aspects of compliance. Each covered entity must designate enough people, depending on the size of the organization, with the responsibility of overseeing various segments of HIPAA compliance (HIPAA Readiness Checklist, 2003). These segments may include a representative from:

❖ Health Information Management Department (Medical Records)
❖ Medical staff
❖ Information technology
❖ Legal advisory
❖ Patient accounts (business office)
❖ Risk management
❖ Satellite clinics
❖ Ancillary departments such as social workers and chaplains

The HIPAA Officer should have an understanding of the scope of the ruling and how each department will be affected. This officer will need to keep abreast of any changes implemented to the ruling in the future.

Depending on the size of the organization, there may be several officers. One person must be designated Security Officer to safeguard the security of the clinical records of patients. The HIPAA Officer may also serve in this capacity. A Privacy Officer must also be designated. This person keeps track of who has access to protected health information. In a small office where one person may have many responsibilities, the functions of the various officers may be fulfilled by as few as two people, using one for backup.

Sufficient access and information must be allowed to provide each employee the information needed to perform their job. The idea of **minimum necessary** is an important concept to understand. Minimum necessary requires that a reasonable effort must be made to limit access to protected health information (PHI) only to what is necessary to accomplish the intended purposes of the use, disclosure, or request.

How much does the receptionist really **need to know** about a patient to keep the appointment schedule, manage the waiting area, and answer the phone? The receptionist will need training to understand when conversations with a patient should be turned over to a nurse, doctor, nurse-practitioner, or other clinical person. The concept of "need to know" is defined as the security principle stating that a user should have access only to the data she needs to perform a particular function. The Privacy Ruling does not limit physicians and nursing staff access to a patient's complete medical record if they need the access to provide care. The ruling is not written to change the manner in which caregivers have accessed medical records in the past. There is to be no limitation on access that would in any way endanger the health or delay the care of any patient. Other people who access PHI have other "need to know" requirements. The information accessed must fit the needs of the job description and nothing more. Persons processing a health claim do not need the same information a certified nursing assistant needs when treating a patient in a long-term care facility. Employees should be *very careful* to not discuss PHI with those outside the scope of their work so that PHI is not disclosed to those who do *not need to know.*

LOCATING THE LATEST TITLE II RULES AND CHANGES

One responsibility of the HIPAA Officer is keeping abreast of any changes in the ruling. Medical journals and periodicals are important sources of information. Perhaps the best way to keep up to date is to use the several websites available provided by the DHHS. The following are websites that will provide good sources of information. It is possible to be on a "listserv" to receive updates and e-mail notices of changes.

1. Subscribe to HIPAA REGS listserv for notification via e-mail of all postings on the final rules at www.cms.hhs.gov/hipaa/hipaa2/regulations/lsnotify.asp. Access the CMS website and navigate to HIPAA and "listservice" enrollment.
2. Centers for Medicare and Medicaid Services at www.cms.gov/hipaa/. This is a government site focusing on Medicare and Medicaid services and issues. It is also a good source of HIPAA information.
3. Government Printing Office for Federal Register documents and original source documents at www.access.gpo.gov/su_docs/fedreg. These documents can be long and confusing. The complete Congressional Record can be accessed here. Summaries are also available.
4. HIPAA guidelines from the (OCR) within the DHHS at www.hhs.gov/ocr/hipaa/guidelines. The OCR is given the responsibility of overseeing the compliance to the HIPAA rulings. This site gives anyone the opportunity to ask questions concerning the rulings. Many questions with accompanying official answers are already posted at this site. Search by topic to see if your question has already been asked.
5. Email questions to askhipaa@cms.hhs.gov. This is the website for the Centers for Medicare and Medicaid Services (CMS).
6. In addition to websites, current information can be obtained by phoning the CMS HIPAA HOTLINE: 1-866-282-0659 (HIPAA Electronic Transaction and Code Sets, 2003).

Appendix A has a listing of the CMS Regional Offices as well as other sources. A number of health organizations conduct seminars to help interpret rulings and any revisions of the rulings. Local seminars will help you connect with others in your field. Networking and sharing of ideas with other health care providers is another valuable source of ideas.

WHAT IS PROTECTED HEALTH INFORMATION?

An efficient way to determine if health information is to be protected is to consider if there is an *association between the health condition and the individual.* If a name or other identifier can be connected with a health condition, diagnosis, or financial status, then that information comes under the HIPAA Privacy Rule and must be protected. The long definition for **protected health information (PHI)** is all *individually identifiable health information* held or transmitted by or to a covered entity in any form or media, whether electronic, paper, or oral. A good understanding of what PHI encompasses will greatly help to understand when disclosure needs to be authorized. PHI is any identifiable health information whether oral, recorded on paper or electronic, any physical or mental health information, a description of services rendered, payment for those services, and personal information that connects the patient to the records. PHI may be a name, an address, a diagnosis, a social security number or other identification number, an insurance policy number, a procedure, or any **psychotherapy notes**. (Handling of these notes needs clarification and a complete explanation will follow later in this chapter.) Any element listed by itself is *not* PHI. A diagnosis alone, an insurance account number alone, or a name alone does not fulfill this definition of PHI. General information that cannot be linked to a particular person does not fulfill this definition. A caregiver is permitted to release a patient's location and general condition. For example, "She is in ICU in critical condition," is permitted. Not permitted is the information that she was taken to ICU because her diabetes became acute.

HIPAA sets a minimum standard for privacy. Personal identifiers of any kind are the targets of identity thefts today. HIPAA law does not address this issue. Every health care provider needs to carefully protect *all* personal information to prevent any opportunity for loss, theft, or unauthorized alteration. Each organization must have policies in place that address the protection of all personal information.

There are subtle ways in which PHI can be disclosed. A location in a nursing home may indicate that a group of rooms are for Alzheimer's patients only, or hospital rooms that are only allotted to patients who are HIV positive. If patient names are displayed on these rooms, you have disclosed PHI. The definition of **disclosure of protected health information** (PHI) is the release, transfer, divulging of, or providing access to PHI to an *outside entity*. This is different from **use** of PHI. The use of PHI is the sharing, employment, application, utilization, examination, or analysis of IIHI *within an entity* that maintains such information. The main difference between these definitions is where the information will end up—inside or outside the covered entity.

PHI is more than electronically transmitted health information. The entire health record of any patient is covered. Included as PHI is radiology film with reports of ultrasounds, Magnetic Resonance Imaging (MRI), Computerized Axial Tomography (CAT scans), tracings or tape printouts from stress tests, any laboratory reports, video tapes of the patient, audio reports or notes, rehabilitation department notes, dictation tapes, nurse's notes, nursing home files, and home health and public health nurse records. PHI may be held by a variety of health care providers. The list may include dentists, chiropractors, optometrists, opticians, morticians, school nurses, nursing homes, home health offices, clinics, and hospitals.

Individually identifiable health information (IIHI) is any demographic information about an individual that can possibly identify that individual. This could be a full or partial name, address, social security number, birth date, or phone number. It can also include a description of someone's past, present, or future physical or mental health or condition; or past, present, or future payment for providing health care to an individual. In some cases, a zip code is an identifier. If all identification is eliminated from the record, and tracing of the individual is not possible, then the HIPAA ruling calls this **de-identified health information.** The best way to de-identify information is to remove all specified identifiers of the individual as well as any information concerning an individual's relatives, household members, and employers. Once this is done, then chances of knowing who the specific individual is will be rare.

Authorization Versus Consent

We have talked about authorization. What does authorization mean? How does it differ from the definition of consent? **Consent** may be needed for *treatment, payment, and normal business operations* and does not need to be written. The patient who comes into a doctor's office and asks for treatment is giving implied consent for treatment. Some providers use the term consent to mean permission to treat. Consent as defined by HIPAA documents is more than agreement to receive treatment. It gives permission to reveal PHI to other health care providers or covered entities in the process of comprehensive treatment, payment of services, and normal health care operations. This is referred to as TPO—treatment, payment, and operations. Long before HIPAA rulings providers asked patients to sign a release of information statement that permits the provider to share information in order to process a claim. HIPAA does not regulate the use of consent for treatment. The regulation of consent was removed from the final rule.

Authorization gives permission to disclose PHI for *reasons other than treatment, payment, or health care operations.* Authorization must include several very specific elements. Authorization for disclosure of PHI must be in writing. It must be in plain language. Authorization gives the covered entity permission to reveal specified health care information or a **designated record set.** The designated record set carefully describes the extent of information to be released. Examples are a doctor's progress notes for a specified date range, a radiology report and film taken on a certain date, or a complete medical record for the past three years. Authorization names the covered entity authorized to disclose the information and the name of the entity or person to receive the information. The purpose of the disclosure is given and expiration of the permission is stated. Proper authorization includes a statement of the individual's right to revoke the authorization and reference to the covered entity's Notice of Privacy Practices that includes that information. Another element to include is the option the covered entity has to condition treatment, payment, or enrollment as a consequence of refusal to sign the authorization. Authorizations must include a statement that the information may be subject to re-disclosure by the recipient, and is therefore no longer protected by federal law. Finally, it must be signed by the individual or their legal representative and dated. An office worker should verify the identity of the individual requesting the release of information, preferably by photo identification.

Health plans have information about the enrollment, payment, claims adjudication, and case or medical management record systems for the individuals covered by their plan. This information, not part of the health care provider's medical records, may only be disclosed with proper authorization. Table 2-1 shows the differences between consent and authorization.

Protected Health Information Concerns and Disclosures

The purpose of the Privacy Rule is to define and limit the circumstances in which an individual's PHI may be used or disclosed by covered entities (OCR Privacy Rule Summary, 2003). Covered entities are required to disclose PHI when individuals specifically request access to it or the DHHS is undertaking a compliance investigation or review. It is noteworthy to understand that the OCR will investigate any complaint received. However, unless the infraction is considered serious, the intent of the investigation will be to correct and adjust policies and procedures so that compliance with the ruling is achieved.

TABLE 2-1 DIFFERENCES BETWEEN CONSENT AND AUTHORIZATION

	Consent	Authorization
Purpose	For TPO (treatment, payment, and health care operations)	For other than TPO
Required by HIPAA	No	Yes
Written	Determined by health care provider policy	Yes, signed and dated

Required Disclosures

The HIPAA ruling requires covered entities to disclose PHI under *two conditions*. The first is when an individual requests access to their medical records. The second required disclosure is when the DHHS comes to review records in regard to a compliance investigation. All other situations have limitations of various types. In most states disclosure in a case of suspected neglect, abuse, or domestic violence is mandatory. This disclosure is listed as disclosure for public interest and to benefit the public and does not need authorization.

Permitted Use and Disclosure Without Authorization

The Privacy Ruling allows six circumstances for permitted use and disclosure of health information *without authorization*. These are as follows:

1. To the individual whose health information it is
2. For treatment, payment, and health care operations
3. With an opportunity to agree or object to inclusion in directory and to disclosure to specified family members
4. Incidental to a permitted use and disclosure
5. For public interest and to benefit the public
6. For research and public health purposes without the identifiable information

For Individual Access.   *Individuals* wishing to see their medical records are permitted to have access to the medical information about them. These include parents, guardians, or other persons acting *in loco parentis* with legal authority to make health care decisions on behalf of the minor children. Certain individuals may designate a "personal representative." This person legally "stands in the shoes" of the individual and has the power to authorize disclosures of health information as well (Personal Representatives, 2002). When someone else is authorized to act for the patient there are rules determining who that person can be and to what extent they can function. Table 2-2 shows how to recognize the personal representative in each category.

For Treatment, Payment, and Health Care Operations.   The second permitted use and disclosure of PHI that does not require authorization is for *treatment, payment, and health care operations*. Broad permission includes any and all services provided by one or more health care providers. This area is where most of the PHI flows just as it did prior to HIPAA mandates. Doctors may share information concerning treatment and care of a patient when referred to another physician. Any procedures of a health plan to obtain premiums, pay claims, and fulfill the responsibilities of the insurance policy are permitted. Permitted health care operations may include quality review by a clinic, hospital, or group of doctors to ensure the best care for each patient; conducting of medical reviews, audits, and legal services; business planning and management; and also certain fundraising activities of the business. An exception: Most psychotherapy notes for treatment and payment as well as health care operations require an authorization *prior to* disclosure. Psychotherapy notes must be treated specially. We address this later in the chapter.

When Permission to Disclose is Obtained.   The third permitted use and disclosure of PHI is when *an individual is asked outright for authorization* to disclose certain information. When

TABLE 2-2 PERSONAL REPRESENTATIVE DEFINITIONS FOR VARIOUS SITUATIONS

If the Individual is: An adult or an *emancipated minor* legal	**The Personal Representative is:** A person with legal authority to make health care decisions on behalf of the individual.	**Example:** Health care power of attorney, court-appointed guardian, general power of attorney.
If the Individual is: An un-emancipated minor	**The Personal Representative is:** A parent, guardian, or other person acting *in loco parentis* with legal authority to make health care decisions on behalf of the minor child.	**Example:** Parent of a minor child, guardian of a minor child, or personal representative of a minor child. Certain exceptions apply—see Limiting Uses/Disclosures.
If the Individual is: Deceased	**The Personal Representative is:** A person with legal authority to act on behalf of the decedent or the estate (not restricted to health care decisions).	**Example:** Executor of the estate, next of kin or other family member, durable power of attorney.

Note: an **emancipated minor** is someone under the age of eighteen (18) who lives independently and is totally self-supporting.

patients are admitted to a hospital facility, it is now practice to ask if the patient would allow contact information to be listed in the facility directory. Under the Privacy Rule, a provider may disclose the individual's general condition and their location within the facility to anyone who requests information *by name*. Often informal permission is granted to allow family and friends to be told the condition and location of a patient when asked for by name. It must be documented that this disclosure occurred with the verbal permission of the patient. That does not allow for a caller to ask for "Somebody, I think his last name is Maxwell." They must give a complete name in order for information to be disclosed. When answering a phone call, one cannot prove that a caller is who they say they are. Medical office personnel are required to make every reasonable effort to verify the identity of the inquirer. Be sure to document the request and the verification effort. When a visitor arrives in person, ask for some identification, preferably a photo ID. This permission is somewhat informal and is considered *what is reasonable* but still protects the patient's privacy. This informal permission also allows a pharmacist to dispense prescriptions to a person acting on behalf of the patient.

Clergy, and clergy only, may be told the religious affiliation of patients with this authorization. It is permitted for clergy members to be told the patients' names who have listed their religious affiliation if it is the same as the clergy member's. For example, a Methodist clergyman is permitted to view the list of patients whose religious affiliation is also listed as Methodist unless the patients have chosen not to be listed in the facility directory.

Disclosures that are Incidental. **Incidental disclosures** are the fourth permitted use of PHI. There will be times when there may be a disclosure of IIHI. When this occurs as a result of or as "incident to" otherwise permitted use or disclosure it is considered incidental. Reasonable safeguards must be in place to prevent this type of disclosure from happening regularly, but if it happens incidentally, there will be no penalty. For example, if a doctor is talking to a patient privately but the conversation is overheard in spite of precautions like closing the door, the disclosure is considered *incidental*.

Disclosures for Public Interest or to Benefit the Public.   There are many disclosure possibilities allowed under the *public interest or to benefit the public* disclosure permit. Briefly, there are 12 national priority purposes for disclosure without an individual's authorization.

1. As *required by law* under specific state law or when ordered by the court.
2. To *control/prevent disease, injury, or disability by public health authorities*. These include communicable diseases and work related illnesses or accidents. This allows public health authorities to monitor trends.
3. In reporting *victims of abuse, neglect, or domestic violence*. The Privacy Rule states that when a physician or other medical care provider reasonably believes that the individual, *whether an unemancipated minor or not*, has been subject to domestic violence, abuse, or neglect by the parent or personal representative, the health care provider may exercise professional judgment and *not* disclose certain health information to them. This follows standards that many states already have in place. The ruling brings a national standard to the issue of releasing PHI in domestic violence, abuse, or neglect cases. A health care provider is legally responsible for reporting such cases to the appropriate authority. This might be the social services department of a local government. The police department is legally responsible when there is a possibility of criminal action. Whether or not the parent or family member is permitted to receive reports of health information is then up to the agency handling the case.
4. For *health oversight activities* such as audits and investigations for oversight of the health care system and government benefit programs.
5. When requested by a *judicial or administrative tribunal* or a subpoena from the courts.
6. For *law enforcement* purposes to identify a suspect or missing person; for information about a victim or suspect; to alert law enforcement of a person's death if the death is suspected to be the result of a criminal act; when PHI is evidence of a crime or assists in law enforcement investigations.
7. Information such as identification of the deceased or to determine the *cause of death* may be disclosed to funeral directors or coroners.
8. PHI may be used to facilitate *donation and transplantation of organs, eyes, or tissue from deceased donors*.
9. When an Institutional Review Board (IRB) or similar organization approves *research*, PHI may be released under strict guidelines. The guidelines limit the usage strictly to research purposes. It is preferable to de-identify research information if possible.
10. If there is believed to be a *serious threat to the health or safety of a person or the public*, covered entities may disclose PHI to civil or law enforcement authorities.
11. Certain *essential governmental functions* have authority to receive PHI. These instances may include assuring proper execution of a military mission, providing protective services to the President, and protecting the health and safety of inmates or employees of a correctional institution.
12. *Workers' compensation laws* and other similar programs have permission to receive an individual's PHI in regard to work-related injuries or illnesses.

Disclosures for Research. Finally the disclosure of PHI is permitted when a **limited data set** has been *de-identified for research purposes*. A limited data set is PHI from which certain specified direct identifiers of individuals and their relatives, household members, and employers have been removed. In other words, de-identified health information may be used for research or for public health purposes with the understanding that specific safeguards are in place so the information cannot be tied to any individual. This may include removing zip codes of areas with a population of less than 10,000 people.

Permitted Use and Disclosure With Authorization

Federal ruling has specified two situations when it is permitted to disclose PHI if given proper authorization. One instance is for notes taken by a psychotherapist. The other permitted use is for purposes of marketing. The medical information shared within the confines of the psychotherapist's office needs special consideration to ensure the parties included have a clear understanding of what the government permits and what must be protected. Many businesses wish to market their products to potential customers. The proper use of PHI for marketing purposes is outlined carefully in the Privacy Ruling.

Disclosure of Psychotherapy Notes. The exceptions listed above do not cover psychotherapy notes. Concerning psychotherapy notes, many states already have regulations that limit their release. Again, the HIPAA Privacy Ruling supplements those regulations and limits disclosing any notes or health information under this category. Special authorization is needed unless the information is to be used for treatment, payment, or health care operations.

The DHHS has issued clarifications concerning the definition of psychotherapy notes. These are more often referred to as *process notes*. They capture the therapist's impressions about the patient. They often contain details considered to be inappropriate for the medical record. These process notes are kept separate within the medical office in order to limit access even in an electronic records system (Psychotherapy Notes, 2000). However, summary information, such as the current state of the patient, medication prescription and monitoring, side effects, counseling sessions start and stop times, modalities and frequencies of treatment furnished, results of clinical tests, and any summary of the following items: diagnosis, functional status, treatment plan, symptoms, prognosis and progress to date, and any other information necessary for treatment or payment, is always placed in the patient's medical record (OCR Privacy Rule Summary, 2003). Summary information is routinely sent to insurers for payment purposes and is treated as PHI.

Psychotherapy notes may be used within the covered entity for management in the treatment of their patient. A covered entity may also defend itself legally and use PHI in its defense. Psychotherapy notes can be used by the DHHS to investigate compliance with the Privacy Rule. Disclosure that is permitted under HIPAA occurs when there appears to be a serious or imminent threat to public health or safely. In this case, health information can be made known to the appropriate authorities in order to protect the individual or the general population.

Disclosure for Marketing Purposes. The Privacy Rule allows for PHI to be used in certain cases for **marketing** purposes. When a marketing arrangement is made between two parties, there is an exchange of direct or indirect payment. Office or hospital workers may ask a patient in person if they may speak to them about some promotional gifts or products they recommend.

If verbal permission is granted, it is considered authorization and should be documented. Otherwise PHI cannot be released for marketing purposes with these four exceptions:

1. You may receive information about health-related products or services that are included in an insurance coverage.
2. Communication about enhancements to a health insurance plan or related services to add to your coverage may be directed to a member of the health plan.
3. A health care provider may communicate various options for treatment to an individual.
4. Communication for case management and coordination of a patient. In addition information given to an individual concerning alternative treatments, therapies, or care settings (such as temporary rehabilitation facilities).

There are several scenarios included at the end of the chapter to help clarify marketing uses.

Limiting Uses and Disclosures

Certain exceptions to the Privacy Ruling apply to parents and un-emancipated minors. The Privacy Rule prohibits a health care provider from disclosing a minor child's PHI when and to the extent that it is expressly prohibited under state or other laws. The Privacy Rule lists three circumstances when PHI is to be withheld from the parent of an un-emancipated minor. The three exceptions are:

1. When a state or other law does not require parental consent and the minor consents to the heath care service. In this instance the Privacy Rule states that parents do not have the right to certain health information.
2. When a court determines that someone other than the parent is allowed to make decisions concerning the medical treatment of a minor.
3. When a parent agrees to a confidential relationship between the minor and the physician. In this situation, if the physician asks the parent(s) if she can speak confidentially with an adolescent child about a medical condition and the parent(s) agree, then that information is restricted from the parents (OCR HIPAA Privacy, 2003).

Minimum Necessary Uses

In all of these situations the Privacy Rule holds to the premise that one may disclose only the "minimum necessary" PHI. A complete record of a patient would be too much information and would not be authorized for most purposes. However, there are exceptions for treatment of a patient by a health care provider, when disclosure is requested by the patient or their personal representative. This includes disclosure to the DHHS for investigation of a complaint, or as required by HIPAA law or other state or local laws. For example, a doctor providing care to a patient is able to access the patient's complete medical records on demand.

In order to comply with the HIPAA ruling, any covered entity must develop a list of persons within their workforce who have complete access to PHI, who have limited access, and *the extent of that access.* It is expected that each office know the *minimum necessary* information for each position within the office workforce. The HIPAA Privacy Officer is the person that oversees this aspect of compliance. She is to provide safeguards that limit the access as outlined. A receptionist would need certain information in order to schedule appointments and understand the time needed for each patient's appointment. The receptionist does not need to know details or have access to the progress notes made for each patient. That information, however, is important for the nursing staff, the doctor, and the coding person in the office. The medical office assistant who does the billing will not need to see the complete medical record. When a claim is in question due to medical necessity the claim should be referred to those individuals who have access to the complete information for adjustments.

BUSINESS ASSOCIATES UNDER PRIVACY RULING

A definition that is important here is **Business Associate (BA).** The Privacy Rule defines Business Associate as a person or organization that performs or assists a function or activity on behalf of a covered entity, but is not part of the covered entity's workforce. Functions may involve the use or disclosure of PHI, including claims processing, data analysis, processing or administration, utilization review, quality assurance, billing, benefit management, practice management, and re-pricing, or someone who provides legal, actuarial, accounting, consulting, accreditation, or financial service to or for a covered entity. A BA can also be a covered entity in its own right.

People or organizations that are BA are those who do not have direct contact with the patient or PHI but who access PHI incidentally in order to do their job. These jobs might include processing insurance claims or servicing copiers. It would also include those doing the coding for claims or fixing a biometric device containing PHI. Transcriptionists, working as contractors, are BA as are the legal advisors for a doctor, clinic, or hospital. These people are not involved with patient care yet are necessary to run the business aspects of the organization. Another category of BA are the vendors who provide equipment and supplies to the covered entity. A copy machine repairman should not be directly exposed to PHI, but she might have access and be unattended. A BA agreement with the copier repair vendor will protect the health care provider.

TRAINING OF THE WORKFORCE AND THE PUBLIC

When April 14, 2003, arrived all medical offices, hospitals, clinics, eye doctors, chiropractors, specialists, and anyone who has records of any health information were required by the Privacy Rule to provide all patients with Notice Of Privacy Practices (NOPP). There are six elements each office must disclose to their patients:

1. The ways they use and disclose PHI
2. Their duties to protect a patient's privacy
3. A notice of their practices to ensure a patient's privacy
4. The terms of the current notice
5. Individual rights concerning PHI
6. A means of contacting the office for further information or to file a complaint (OCR Privacy Rule Summary, 2003)

Since April 14, 2003, every health care provider who makes direct face-to-face contact with a patient is required to obtain from the patient a written acknowledgment of the receipt of these privacy notices. The NOPP cannot be summarized and offered to the patient. The disclosure of NOPP *must* be complete. A signed receipt of the NOPP must be in a patient's record.

The Privacy Rule gives patients a right to access their medical records. They can obtain a copy of their records. The original belongs to the agent or medical office that created them. Simply because a name is on the records does not mean that person has complete claim to all the papers or other ancillary records. This ruling also gives anyone the right to *amend* her medical record by appending it. This is an addition to, not a change of, their record. If a patient disagrees with something in her record, she may add to the record written comments or other documentation of her choosing. A patient may add information that she feels is missing. However, a covered entity has the option to deny this request to amend the record. In this case the individual is permitted to submit a statement of disagreement and have that statement of disagreement included in the medical record. This option of viewing and possibly amending one's medical record is not a new procedure. The federal government has now made a uniform ruling about how this can be done in any state.

The Privacy Rule also allows a patient the option of restricting who receives access to their PHI. Individuals have the right to see a listing of who has accessed their records and what has been disclosed. This listing does not include disclosures for treatment, payment, and health care operations (TPO), which are normal and routine operations necessary to conduct business.

The DHHS understands that the Privacy Rule must be flexible to meet all sizes of covered entities. The ruling is written so that each provider can implement the Privacy Rule to meet the needs of its own particular situation. The Department *does expect* each provider to have: (1) written policy and procedures; (2) a Privacy Official within the organization; (3) a workforce that is trained to comply with the ruling. Everyone employed is expected to know where to find the privacy policies of that office. They may be written and kept current in a policy book located in the office. The policies may be available electronically through intranet or Internet access rather than on paper. The workers are also expected to understand how the policies affect their particular areas of work. An important expectation of the DHHS is that a provider may not retaliate against a person for exercising her rights. Each organization must have appropriate safeguards in place to prevent inappropriate disclosure of PHI and a means to relieve or resolve any harmful effect that might be caused if an inappropriate disclosure of PHI has occurred. Each covered entity must maintain its privacy policies and procedures for at least six years after their creation.

ENFORCEMENT GUIDELINES

The main intent of those guidelines is *not* to criminally punish or impose fines. Strong enforcement from the OCR will be evident when there is blatant and obvious disregard for the ruling and resistance to correcting the problem. Noncompliance with the Privacy Rule does bring civil penalties and possible criminal penalties if the violation is severe. The DHHS seeks to foster cooperation with the ruling rather than impose penalties. However, if failure to comply is found, then the following penalties may be imposed. A penalty of $100 per incidence may be imposed. Multiple violations in a calendar year may not exceed $25,000 per year. When the

OCR finds a person knowingly obtains or discloses PHI, a fine of $50,000 and imprisonment up to one year may be imposed. These criminal penalties may be increased to $100,000 and up to five years' imprisonment if the wrongful conduct involves false pretenses, and up to $250,000 and ten years' imprisonment if the conduct involves the intent to sell, transfer, or use IIHI for commercial advantage, personal gain, or malicious harm. These sanctions will be enforced by the Department of Justice (OCR Privacy Rule Summary, 2003).

These penalties notwithstanding, it is the position of the DHHS that they strive to assist organizations to comply with the ruling. They do not want to prosecute. Their goal is to enable the system to work. As long as they find a willingness to adjust and correct situations, then enforcement will be a helpful, not a dreadful thing.

SUMMARY

The Privacy Ruling written by the DHHS creates standards for protecting all IIHI in the country. Implementation began in April 2003 for all health care providers. It allows health care providers to access information to fully and adequately treat their patients. Each provider must have policies in place to comply with the Privacy Ruling. The ruling allows each office to comply in a manner that is "reasonable" for their particular setting.

Each covered entity must have someone designated to oversee this compliance—the HIPAA Officer. Depending upon the size of the entity, this may be a single person or a committee. The officer or committee is responsible for overseeing the training of all workers and for keeping abreast of any updates by the DHHS. Changes in rulings can be accessed easily through Internet access to the DHHS website.

The Privacy Rule applies to all covered entities. The focus is to ensure the privacy of PHI. Information designated as PHI is determined if there can be an association between a personal identifier and a health condition.

Authorization is granted to disclose PHI for a specific purpose. Authorization states what is to be disclosed, to whom it is to be disclosed, and when the authorization expires. There are exceptions when dealing with parents and minor children. In any suspected case of domestic violence, abuse, or neglect, disclosure to authorities is mandatory.

Psychotherapy notes require specific authorization from the patient even if disclosure is for TPO. All staff is to have access to the "minimum necessary" amount of PHI that is needed to fulfill their job responsibility. Clinical workers will have the greatest access since they treat the patient directly.

There are several permitted uses or disclosures of PHI without written authorization. The Privacy Rule outlines when use or disclosure is permitted only with written authorization. Some PHI may be used for marketing purposes. The specifics are carefully outlined so individual health information is not distributed outside the scope of the covered entity solely for the purpose of selling a product or service.

Many organizations work alongside health care providers who have access to some or part of PHI as Business Associates. Business Associates agree to protect all health information they may encounter in their business dealings.

The Privacy Rule directed all providers to provide every patient with a NOPP. This outlines how their PHI will be used and protected, and how the patient can contact the provider if there is a problem or complaint. Penalties and criminal charges are outlined when the OCR investigates. If the OCR finds non-compliance and unwillingness toward compliance, they have the obligation to impose penalties in the form of fines and possibly criminal charges.

END OF CHAPTER QUESTIONS

1. What does the term "covered entity" mean? What are the three categories of *covered entities*? Are all physician offices covered entities?

2. Do insurance companies who provide automobile and life insurance fall under the HIPAA ruling?

3. A medical office does not use electronic means to send their insurance claims. Are they considered a *covered entity?*

4. Which five departmental areas must the HIPAA Officer contact in order to train them to be compliant with the HIPAA ruling?

5. What is protected health information?

6. Explain what is meant by minimum necessary.

7. How might a medical office *de-identify* health information?

8. An authorization has an expiration date. How does this protect privacy?

9. Who might be the "personal representative" for: an emancipated minor? an un-emancipated minor? a deceased person?

10. List eight examples of disclosure of PHI for the benefit of the public.

11. Why is it important that the HIPAA Privacy Ruling cover *Business Associates?*

12. Who in the health care organization is responsible for knowing where the written policies regarding HIPAA compliance are located?

13. What government department investigates complaints about the HIPAA Ruling?

14. What type of attitude does the OCR expect to find when investigating a health care facility?

15. What is the minimum penalty that the OCR may impose for failure to comply with the HIPAA Ruling?

Scenarios

How would you answer?

1. As receptionist for a physician, you call a patient to remind them of an upcoming appointment. No one answers the phone and you are directed to leave a voice message. What can you say?

2. Are postcard reminders legal under HIPAA?

3. To prevent patients from overhearing discussions with a doctor, must all examining rooms be soundproofed?

4. A hospital uses PHI about an individual to provide health care to the individual and then consults with other health care providers about the individual's treatment. Is authorization needed?

5. A psychoanalyst forwards a patient's health care information to another health care provider for further treatment by that provider. Is authorization needed?

6. A hospital sends a patient's health care instructions to a nursing home to which the patient is being transferred. Is authorization needed?

7. A contract computer repairperson asks for the logon and password to test a computer. May she have access because she has signed a Business Associate contract?

8. Several thousand patient records at the University of Michigan Medical Center inadvertently lingered on a public Internet site for two months. The problem was discovered when a student searching for information about a doctor was linked to files containing private patient records with names, addresses, phone and Social Security numbers, job status, treatments for medical conditions, and other data (Black Eye at the Med Center, 1999). How does HIPAA address this problem?

9. An advertisement is received from a hospital informing former patients about a new cardiac facility, which is not part of the hospital, that can provide a baseline EKG for $39. The communication is not for the purpose of providing treatment advice. Is this considered marketing?

10. A hospital uses its patient list to announce the arrival of a new specialty group (e.g., orthopedic) or the acquisition of new equipment (e.g., x-ray machine) through a general mailing or publication. Is this considered marketing?

11. A primary care physician refers an individual to a specialist for a follow-up test or provides free samples of a prescription drug to a patient. Is this considered marketing?

12. A hospital provides a free package of formula and other baby products to new mothers as they leave the maternity ward. Is this considered marketing?

See Appendix C for more scenario questions.

REFERENCES

Black eye at the med center. (1999, February 22). *Washington Business.*

Crowley, S. (2000, March). Invading your medical privacy. *AARP Bulletin*, p. 1.

Hillig, T., & Mannies, J. (2001, July 3). Woman sues over posting of abortion details. *St. Louis Post-Dispatch*, p. A1.

HIPAA electronic transaction and code sets. (2003, March). Volume 1, Paper 1, Centers for Medicare and Medicaid Services, p. 1.

HIPAA Readiness Checklist. (2003, March). Provider HIPAA checklist, moving toward compliance. *CMS/HIPAA Electronic Transactions and Code Sets.* p. 1.

Office of civil rights privacy rule summary. (2003, April). Summary of the HIPAA Privacy Rule, p. 4.

Personal representatives OCR HIPAA privacy. (2002, December 3, revised April 3, 2003). (codified at 45CFR164.502(g)). p. 1.

Psychotherapy Notes, Standards for Privacy of Individually Identifiable Health Information No. 250, 65 Fed. Reg., 82622-23 (2000, December 28).

Transactions and Code Sets

CHAPTER OUTLINE

Introduction

Purpose of Transaction Standards

Designated Code Sets

    Diagnosis Codes

    Inpatient Procedure Codes

    Outpatient Procedure Codes

    Dental Procedure Codes

    Drug Codes

    Non-medical Code Sets

ASC X12 Nomenclature

    Data Overview

    Architecture

    Use of Loops

    Sample of EDI Claim Data

Limitations to Claims Encounters

Remittance Advice and Secondary Payer

Working With Outside Entities

    Trading Partner Agreements

    Business Use and Definition

Summary

KEY TERMS

adjudication

ASC X12

biologic

code set

crossover claim

Electronic Data Interchange (EDI)

etiology

format

HCPCS—**H**ealth [**C**are Financing
Administration] **C**ommon **P**rocedure
Coding **S**ystem

nomenclature

orthotic

protocol

Provider Taxonomy Code

subscriber

Trading Partner

Trading Partner Agreement (TPA)

X12N

THINK ABOUT IT

1. Computer language is like reading a foreign language. Do I need to learn this language to understand Electronic Data Interchange (EDI) transactions?

2. What happens if a transaction file arrives at the wrong destination?

3. Is the whole transmission spoiled if a single digit is transposed?

4. Will the payer tell you what is wrong with your transmission?

INTRODUCTION

The next federal mandate concerning the flow of health care information takes the form of electronic transmission of protected health information (PHI). In order for all parties to communicate efficiently a standard must be defined so each health plan, health care provider, and health care clearinghouse can communicate to each other. In other words, all parties must adopt a common language. The Department of Health and Human Services (DHHS) looked to standards developed in the business world. The DHHS found that the Accredited Standards Committee (ASC) had developed standards that have been tested and found secure for use in most other industries. The next step was to define the language to use in electronic health care transactions and the form or architecture of these transactions. The Standards for Electronic Transactions became effective on October 16, 2000. An extension was later added and the implementation date was moved to October 16, 2003. A final rule titled *Modifications to Electronic Data Transaction Standards and Code Sets* was printed in the Federal Register on February 20, 2003. Some compliance exceptions were permitted until a final date of October 16, 2004.

Any transaction of PHI between any of the three covered entities must be translated into the federal standard. This was good news for the health care provider since the different varieties of claim forms disappeared. It also brought a problem for the health plans that wanted certain other types of information to better adjudicate (or process) their claims. Explanation of the various parts of this ruling follows.

PURPOSE OF TRANSACTION STANDARDS

The Transaction and Code Sets portion of HIPAA Administrative Simplification is the centerpiece where promised savings and simplification are realized. With the implementation of this title of the Health Insurance Portability and Accountability Act (HIPAA), health care providers began to see that accounts receivable days diminished, which increased cash flow to their organization. The cost of office overhead also declined. Patients may now know at the time of their visit the exact insurance coverage they are able to receive. These changes elevate the level of confidence conveyed to patients using health care facilities.

The health care industry is the only major industry in the United States that processes the majority of its transactions on paper. It has not seriously considered standardizing transactions handling using Electronic Data Interchange (EDI). Banks, money exchanges, stock exchanges, steel plants, manufacturing plants, and many others conduct business in a secure electronic **format** based on EDI. An electronic format is an arrangement of data elements that assist in identifying the data content of a transaction. Since the use of EDI began, many businesses have streamlined tedious data entry tasks. Because of EDI the overall expense of doing business has shrunk for organizations of all sizes. Congress motivated the health care providers to use a tried and true media.

The administrative simplification provisions of HIPAA law were passed with the support of the health care industry. Only with federal help would all individual providers be able to submit transactions in a uniform way. Individual health plans could not agree on a standard without giving some competitors a market advantage. The HIPAA law levels the playing field for all health plans. It does not require all transactions be submitted electronically, but those that are submitted in that manner are now standardized (Department of Health and Human Services, 2003).

The ASC has developed standards for the cross-industry exchange of electronic business information since the 1980s. By the year 2000, more than 300,000 companies used **Electronic Data Interchange (EDI)** and the ASC X12 system to transmit information. This electronic system is defined as computer-to-computer transmission of business information in a standard format using national standard communications **protocols,** or a set of conventions governing the formatting of data in an electronic communications system. By using this electronic interchange with their business partners, industries have saved billions of dollars in office costs. Businesses have greatly expanded the reach of their markets through this secure and streamlined exchange of data. Note the remarkable efficiencies used extensively in the auto industry that make "just in time" processes work. Inventory is tracked in detail so a minimum of warehouse space is used to store parts.

There are currently more than 300 standards for electronic transactions. HIPAA has initially adopted eight of these standards for use with transmitting protected health information (PHI). There are more standards being considered for adoption. The first of these include *First*

Report of Injury for workers' compensation claims and *Claims Attachments.* The ASC oversees development of all standards. Changes are implemented only after obtaining a consensus of those using the standard. This has benefited the business world for over 25 years. Businesses have seen reduced cycle time of their inventory, increased productivity, reduced costs, improved accuracy, improved business relationships, enhanced customer service, increased sales, minimized paper use and storage, and increased cash flow. Certainly there will be similar benefits to the health care industry as they use **ASC X12 standards**.

EDI allows offices to transmit information without rekeying or other human intervention. Information contained in an EDI transaction set is, for the most part, the same as on conventional documents. The importance to the health care provider and payer is that information will be transmitted via instantaneous electronic means rather than slow-moving paper. The same information required for a paper insurance claim will still be needed. The electronic transmission will be efficient and timesaving. The challenge for the covered entities will be to manage the hardware and software that transmits this information. A typical medical office assistant, doctor, or clinical worker will need to understand the workings of the transaction. They will need to understand who can train them and who can assist them when errors occur.

Parts 160 and 162 of Title II in the HIPAA ruling outlines standards for eight approved electronic transactions and for the **code sets** to be used in those transactions. These eight original forms for electronic communication are to be used exclusively between health plans, health care clearinghouses, and health care providers. This ruling does not eliminate the use of paper claims submitted on HCFA-1500, UB-92, or dental forms. These are still permitted and in some limited cases preferable. In time, even the exceptions will be phased out in favor of the electronic media. Claims made where medical charges require explanation will still need to be submitted on paper along with supporting documentation until the standard for attachments to health claims has been implemented. Planning committees are developing means of explanation to be included within the transaction set so the need for supporting documentation will be reduced. The ruling addresses the use of electronic media to transmit PHI between health plans, health care clearinghouses, and certain health care providers. The definition of "certain health care providers" includes only those who transmit health information in electronic form in connection with a transaction covered by this portion of HIPAA. Only when the change is made to the electronic form does the ruling apply.

Each covered entity needs to manage the transmission of health care information. This means all covered entities such as all private health plans including managed care programs and government health plans such as Medicare, state Medicaid programs, the Military Health care system, the Veterans Health Administration, and the Indian Health Service programs. Any health care clearinghouse and health care provider are also covered entities. There is a certain amount of information you need to know before you can manage EDI. It is not necessary to understand the complete process of electronic transmissions. It is like knowing and using electricity. Most of us understand some basic elements of electricity but complete knowledge of exactly how electricity works is not necessary to use it effectively. A trusted software vendor should be retained who is qualified to implement and support EDI applications. The workforce must have enough understanding to know when to call for outside help. Training should focus on accurate and acceptable transmissions. Questions should first be asked of the software vendor. The Centers for Medicare and Medicaid Services (CMS), who oversee compliance, are another source for help. There should be training for individuals within the organization to properly operate the software and hardware needed to make transmissions secure.

Submitting paper claims is a poor option since it continues to be costly. Another disadvantage is that it extends the accounts payable time in collection of money due the health care provider. The cost of following up with phone calls, printing and mailing billing statements, and eventually having a collection agency contact the patient reduces the actual funds the doctor receives for patient care. Bad debt increases sharply on aging accounts. The initial cost of transition to electronic claim submission means an investment of computer equipment and software to be able to handle the change. Software vendors must adjust their products as the processes are changed. In time we will see the inevitable change to EDI as acceptable, desired, and pervasive.

DESIGNATED CODE SETS

EDI requires certain coding to explain lengthy descriptions. Under HIPAA, a *code set* is any set of codes used for encoding data elements, such as tables of terms, medical concepts, medical diagnoses, or medical procedures. The medical and clinical codes explain the diagnosis, procedure performed, drug used, services rendered, and supplies provided. It standardizes the codes to be used and eliminates any local or health plan issued codes. The HIPAA ruling designates certain sources to be used in coding items such as diagnoses, procedures for outpatients and inpatients, drugs and biologics, and dental procedures. Medicare originates a **Health Care [Financing Administration] Procedure Coding System (HCPCS),** nicknamed "hick-pick." These codes are referred to as Level II codes. Medicare has endorsed the *CPT-4* coding and the HCPCS and often refers to these two systems of procedural codes as HCPCS codes. This part of the ruling does not alter the work of coders very much. In some ways it makes their work easier because the Level III codes that had been used are now eliminated. The other categories of codes are non-medical codes. Some examples are state abbreviations, provider specialty, and remittance remarks to explain adjustments on a remittance. In response to a claim there are several categories of codes used to codify reasons relating to the judgment for or against payment or **adjudication** of the claim. Medical codes pertain to a patient encounter.

Diagnosis Codes

The *International Classification of Diseases, 9th Edition, Clinical Modification,* Volumes 1 and 2 (*ICD-9-CM*) is used to report diseases, injuries, impairments, causes of injury, disease, impairment, or other health-related problems. Volumes 1 and 2 encompass the entire listing of possible diseases, injuries, and impairments. The two volumes include alphabetical and tabular listings. Any other identification system for diagnosis coding is not considered compliant with HIPAA rulings. *ICD-9-CM* is updated yearly. New codes are valid beginning October 1 of each year. However, beginning in 2005, the DHHS will issue revisions twice a year: April 1 and October 1. This change is a result of the Medicare Prescription Drug, Improvement, and Modernization Act of 2003.

It is important to note that the World Health Organization (WHO) revises the *International Classification of Diseases.* The tenth revision has the support of the National Center for Health Statistics and the Health Care Financing Administration, now known as the Centers for Medicare and Medicaid Services (CMS), and the American Health Information Management Association (AHIMA). The clinical modifications have been complete for several years. Once the deadlines for HIPAA compliance are complete, the change to the *ICD-10-CM* diagnosis coding will be the next issue facing the health care industry. These changes for diagnoses and injuries will increase the coding system to four, five, or six spaces using both alpha and numeric identifiers. The tenth revision also includes laterality—which side—within the code itself. Many new understandings of disease and the **etiology** of conditions have changed since 1975 when the ninth classification of diseases was developed. As a result the tenth revision groups some diseases differently from the ninth revision.

Inpatient Procedure Codes

Procedures or other actions taken for diseases, injuries, and impairments performed on *inpatients* are to be coded from Volume 3 of *ICD-9-CM*. This does not change inpatient coding from the prior standard. This volume is used only by hospitals, long-term care facilities, and similar inpatient institutions and for claims on inpatients. These four-digit codes are currently being used by hospitals to report prevention, diagnosis, treatment, and management procedures. This volume is updated yearly, and new codes are valid beginning January 1 of each year. Many publishers provide all three volumes of the *ICD-9-CM* in one text. Many software vendors provide programs for coding that are based on the *ICD-9-CM*. The software asks a series of questions to establish an appropriate coding path. This helps the coder to find the correct code by eliminating all other options.

Another important issue to consider is that just as there has been a move by organizations like AHIMA to incorporate the *ICD-10-CM* diagnosis coding into the United States standards, there is also a similar move to adopt the procedural coding of the *International Classification of Diseases-10th Revision Procedure Coding System (ICD-10-PCS)*. The CMS arranged with 3-M Health Information Systems to develop a comprehensive system of procedural coding to replace the *ICD-9-CM* procedure codes. The *ICD-10-PCS* has been developed to complement the diagnosis system. It is designed in a very different manner from the current *CPT-4* coding system or the Volume 3 *ICD-9-CM* procedures. There are a total of seven characters for each procedure listed. By using both letters and numbers there are a possible 34 different values for each of the seven spaces. The letters "O" and "I" are not used so there is no confusion with the numbers zero and one. This system of coding does not include any diagnostic information, only a procedure and its method of delivery (how it was accomplished).

Outpatient Procedure Codes

Procedure codes for *physician services* and other health-related services are to be found in the *Current Procedural Terminology, 4th Edition (CPT-4)*. This coding system is maintained by the American Medical Association (AMA). These codes are five digits without any decimal. They include Evaluation and Management (E/M) services, anesthesia procedures, surgical procedures, radiology, pathology, and laboratory services as well as services dealing with medicines and their application to the patient. This last section includes psychiatry procedures, ophthalmology procedures, therapeutic cardiovascular services, and therapies of various types among other services. This volume is updated yearly and new codes are valid in January of each year.

The Healthcare Common Procedural Coding System (HCPCS) contains codes for physician services as well as many other *non-physician provided health care services and equipment*. The HCPCS codes are updated annually with new codes becoming valid January 1 of each year and distributed by the DHHS. If services and provisions are *not administered by a physician,* then HCPCS is the place to find that alphanumeric code. The HCPCS codes lists substances, equipment, supplies, and other items used in health care services. These may include items such as ambulance and other transporting services, medical supplies, **orthotic** (a support or brace for weak or ineffective joints or muscles) and prosthetic devices, and durable medical equipment. These codes consist of six characters. The first is a letter followed by five numerals. They are referred to as Level II HCPCS codes.

Over the years, state Medicaid agencies have developed many local codes, Level III codes, to provide clarification of the services rendered to their clients. The HIPAA regulation mandated the adoption of a uniform standard without any local codes. This meant that the 30,000 local codes developed by various state Medicaid programs must be moved into a CPT or HCPCS code. Much negotiating and compromising ensued, with the result that most local codes were moved into current CPT or HCPCS codes and currently accepted modifiers. Workgroup committees eventually detailed 500 recommendations for new codes and/or modifiers to be adopted by the *CPT-4* agency—the AMA, or HCPCS developer—the CMS.

The AMA has worked on improving the structure and process of *CPT-4.* These procedures include both inpatient and outpatient procedural coding. Changes in this system, *Current Procedural Terminology-5th Edition* (*CPT-5*), will be minor and include many revised or new codes.

Dental Procedure Codes

Dentists use a separate coding book referred to as *Current Dental Terminology, Version 4.* This is commonly referred to as *CDT-4,* an American Dental Association publication. These are revised biannually starting January 1 of odd-numbered years—2003, 2005, and 2007, for example. There are ten categories of services for dental patients. They include diagnostic services, preventive services, restorative services, endodontics, peridontics, removable prosthodontics, implant services, fixed prosthodontics, oral and maxillofacial surgery, and adjunctive general services. These codes are similar to Common Procedure Coding System (HCPCS Level II) codes in that they begin with the letter D followed by four numerals. The way to distinguish these from the HCPCS code is the beginning letter "D."

Drug Codes

The DHHS designated that drugs are to be coded from the National Drug Code (NDC) System. This listing of drugs was established under the Medicare program. The NDC serves as a universal product identifier for drug reimbursement for retail pharmacy drug transactions. It is updated by the DHHS in collaboration with drug manufacturers. These codes are used by retail pharmacies to list drugs used to fill doctor's prescriptions. This includes both drugs and **biologics**. Biologics are products that are used to make medicines. The codes are unique 10-digit, 3-segment numbers. Each number identifies the labeler/vendor, product, and trade package size. The NDC uses one of the following configurations: 4-4-2, 5-3-2, or 5-4-1. The first segment of the identifier indicates the firm that manufacturers, repackages, or distributes a drug product. The drug manufacturer assigns the product and package numbers—the second and third portions of the code. Drugs listed in the NDC are limited to prescription drugs and a few selected over the counter (OTC) products. Details about any drug can be found at the website for the United States Food and Drug Administration, www.fda.gov.

Non-medical Code Sets

HIPAA defined non-medical code sets used strictly for administrative purposes. These codes do not refer directly to the medical care of a patient. They include items in an insurance claim such as state abbreviations, zip codes, telephone area codes, race, and ethnicity codes. There are code sets developed for use in the electronic transaction to identify the physician's specialty training, payment policies, the status of a claim, why claims have been denied or adjusted, type of health plan, benefits, patient eligibility, provider organization type, disability type, and reasons for rejection, to name a few.

In order to identify the specialty training for a particular doctor, there is a **Provider Taxonomy Code.** The National Uniform Claim Committee (NUCC) Data Subcommittee maintains this set of codes. These codes identify the provider type and area(s) of specialization for each health care provider. As the DHHS develops the physician unique federal identifier, this taxonomy code will be phased out. The new coding system is to be free from identifiers so that the location or specialty of the physician cannot be determined.

There are several other code sets that help explain other functions of the health plan. Example of these non-medical codes are *Claim Adjustment Reason Codes* and *Reject Reason Codes.* These codes explain the payment policies that affect reimbursement.

Another type of code is *Remittance Advice Remark Codes.* When information is lacking or needs further clarification one of these codes is returned to the provider for clarification of the rejection.

Claim Status Codes and *Claim Status Category Codes* communicate to the health care provider a particular claim's status. The category code of "F2" means the claim or line has been denied. Other codes explain in detail the status such as entity is not approved as an electronic submitter, special handling required at health plan site, or duplicate of a previously processed claim/line. These are all examples of non-medical code sets that the DHHS has adopted for the EDI transmissions.

ASC X12 NOMENCLATURE

The American National Standards Institute (ANSI) is recognized worldwide as an authoritative organization in standard setting. This organization is given the authority to develop standards and designate **nomenclatures** or give the standards names that are recognized internationally. The Accredited Standards Committee (ASC) and the DHHS created a new committee—National Uniform Claim Committee (NUCC)—to develop a standardized data set to be implemented for HIPAA transactions formerly sent on the HCFA-1500 form. The National Uniform Claim Committee (NUCC) sets the standards for content and data definitions for non-institutional health care claims in the United States. The standardized data set outlines how and in what order the information is to be sent through EDI in the ASC **X12N** standard to and from third-party payers. The "X12 N" nomenclature designates the EDI standards for the insurance industry. The NUCC consists of representatives from the AMA, the CMS, representatives from key provider and payer organizations, and state and federal regulators. Representatives from both health care providers and health care payers provided input from their industries. Their recommendations complement the work of the Accredited Standards Committee Electronic Date Interchange (ASC X12N) in complying with the HIPAA law.

Washington Publishing Company (WPC) has developed implementation guides for assisting information management technicians to administer and support the X12N transmissions. The "N" transmissions are the transaction standards for the insurance industry. The WPC manages the manufacturing and distribution process and holds the copyright for the X12N Implementation Guides on behalf of the X12N Subcommittee.

Data Overview

To understand a little of what is going through the communication wires in EDI, we will examine some of the terms and concepts of computer communications. Any one transaction set contains groups of logically related data in units called segments. A data element is the smallest named unit of information in the ASC X12 standard. For instance, the N4 segment used in the transaction set conveys the city, state, zip code, and other geographic information. A transaction set contains multiple segments, so the addresses of different parties, for example, can be conveyed from one computer to the other. An analogy would be that the transaction set is like a freight train; the segments are like the train's cars; and each segment can contain several data elements in the same manner that a train car can hold multiple crates (ACS X12N Guide, 2000). The information is sent with a "header" and a "trailer" segment. These tell the computer when to start and end the claim. These markers define the data element separators and terminator. They identify the sender and receiver. The markers provide controls for the interchange and also allow authorization and security for the transmission.

Architecture

The ASC has set up templates or architecture for each of their defined transactions. The WPC is responsible for maintaining and providing Internet access to these standards. Their website is www.wpc-edi.com. The transactions created in the HIPAA ruling are:

1. ASC X12N **837**—Health Care Claim: Dental, Professional, or Institutional
2. ASC X12N **270**—Health Care Eligibility Benefit Inquiry
3. ASC X12N **271**—Health Care Eligibility Benefit Response
4. ASC X12N **276**—Health Care Claim Status Request
5. ASC X12N **277**—Health Care Claim Status Response
6. ASC X12N **278**—Health Care Services Review
7. ASC X12N **834**—Benefit Enrollment and Maintenance
8. ASC X12N **835**—Health Care Claim Payment/Advice

The transaction templates are the first ones accepted by the federal government to send and receive PHI between providers and payers. Medical office personnel do need to understand the details of these transactions. Since HIPAA does not specify how the provider complies, software vendors have provided many options for health care providers to use. It is the health care providers' responsibility that the formats they use comply with HIPAA standards. The software vendor is providing a service to the provider. The ultimate responsibility for accuracy lies with the provider.

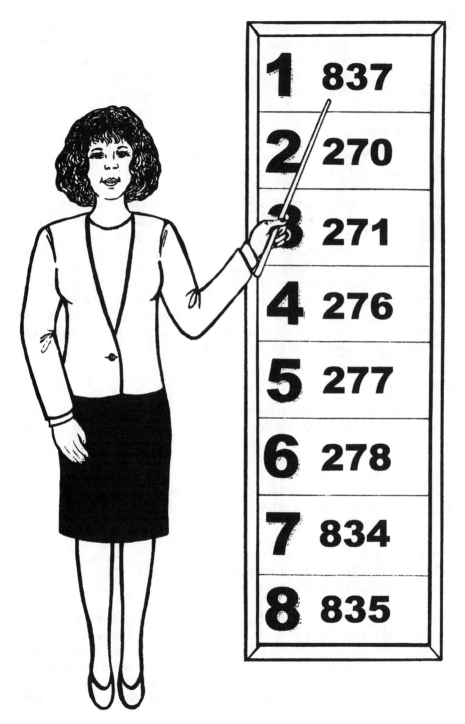

Figure 3-1 In 2003 the Department of Health and Human Services issued these eight transaction formats. More will follow as they are developed.

The following titles are for claim forms:

Health Care Institutional ASC X12N 837, version 4010 X 96
Health Care Dental ASC X12N 837, version 4010 X 097
Health Care Professional ASC X12N 837, version 4010 X 98

There are three versions of the claim form that cover institutional/hospital claims, dental claims, and physician/professional claims. The paper forms for dentists, doctors, and hospitals were different so the electronic format is unique to accommodate these differences. The institutional claim covers hospitals, nursing facilities, and similar inpatient institutions. The professional version is designed for physician services, providers of durable medical equipment, and similar suppliers. In time, as needs change, these transaction standards contain the flexibility to adapt easily in the future.

Health Care Eligibility Benefit Inquiry ASC X12N 270 relates to an inquiry concerning a patient's eligibility for benefits from a health plan or to determine if a specific procedure is covered (eligible for payment) under the patient's policy. The companion form, *Health Care Eligibility Benefit Response* ASC X12N 271, is the standard for reply. The efficiency of an electronic request and reply provides more time for health care providers to take care of patient needs in a timely manner. It also permits physicians to discuss options at the time of treatment with the patient if coverage is denied or only partially covered.

Health Care Claim Status Request ASC X12N 276 requests information about the status of the claim that has been transmitted. The reply uses *Health Care Claim Response* ASC X12N 277 format. A typical code reply may be "P3"—pending/requested information, "F2"—finalized/denial, or "R3"—requests for additional information/claim/line.

Health Care Services Review ASC X12N 278 is the standard for electronic exchange of requests and responses between health care providers and health plans in regard to certification and authorization for procedures. It is standard to receive an authorization number from a health plan and to include that number on the claim form. This helps assure that services will be paid. It can also provide information to the health care provider of how much the plan will pay for specific procedures. This information allows the physician to better assess the best means to treat the patient in question and to advise them of what to expect from their health plan. With secondary and possibly third payers, this request allows the provider to quickly receive information from all parties involved in payment.

This form, *Health Care Services Review/Request* X12N 278, also allows authorization for a patient to be referred to another provider. With many Preferred Provider Organizations (PPO), the options for referrals are limited to a specific list. The primary physician is quickly able to determine if a provider is authorized.

Benefit Enrollment and Maintenance ASC X12N 834 enables health care providers and health plans to exchange individual, **subscriber** (person named as the holder of the insurance policy), and dependent enrollment information. As policies change for particular plans, the health care provider can keep abreast of any changes of the policy. The extent of PHI that can be included in this transaction is limited to the "minimum necessary" for proper response. A health care provider will also be able to receive information concerning "disenrollment" from a health plan. By not paying premiums a patient may be disenrolled from the health plan or a patient may change employment and not continue the same coverage. Medicaid provisions are reviewed monthly by each state agency so eligibility for aid may change on a monthly basis. It is important to request current status so that payment for services can be requested from the patient or guarantor if coverage is suspended or cancelled.

Health Care Claim Payment/Advice ASC X12N 835 is the transaction coming from the health plan with remittance advice, much the same as the coordination of benefits or remittance advice did prior to HIPAA. The transmission includes two pieces of information: the payment containing information about the transfer of funds and the explanation of benefits detailing coverage of billed procedures and services. With electronic banking, providers can receive payments to their bank accounts via electronic transfer. This puts funds into the health care provider's available cash flow almost immediately after services are provided. The explanation of benefits portion of the reply advises the health care provider of any adjustments, deductible amounts for the guarantor to pay, and other pertinent information about payment of the claim.

Use of Loops

The architecture of the file is set up with many different loops. Loops are parts of information taken from the insurance claim form HCFA-1500 for physician and supplier services or UB-92 in the case of inpatient billing. Each loop contains a piece of information needed to complete the claim. As with paper insurance forms, there are more loops than needed every time. Only the loop that has information in it is sent as the data string. The first section is the header. This begins the data string and identifies the "engine," the type of transaction, who is submitting the claim, and who is receiving the claim. The next category gives detailed information about the billing party and information about electronic debiting of the account so payment can be made electronically. Information about the subscriber or insured is then transmitted. Other loops include the patient name and demographic information. The largest loop is the claim detail information. The diagnosis information, procedures performed, and their charges are listed in this loop. Other information is included in this loop such as dates of hospitalization, amount patient has paid on account, authorization numbers, and referral information where applicable. Other loops include information about the attending physician, operating physician, service facility, and other payer information when secondary insurance is available. Finally, there is the "trailer" data, which tells the computer the end of the claim has been reached.

We will look at the information from a sample insurance claim that would be sent by a hospital for a patient. The charges included are for preliminary blood test, CPT-4 code: 85025—hemogram and platelet count, automated, and automated partial differential WBC count, and CPT 4 code: 93005—electrocardiogram, tracing only without interpretation. These are procedures in preparation for cataract surgery. Principal diagnosis is 366.9: Unspecified cataract. Secondary diagnoses are 401.9: Unspecified Essential Hypertension and 794.31: Abnormal Electrocardiogram. The inpatient surgery is *ICD-9-CM, Vol. 3* procedure: 15.3. Operations on two or more extraocular muscles involving temporary detachment from globe, one or both eyes. Here is the information in the traditional UB-92 format on paper. Following is the listing of information included in the data string for the electronic transmission.

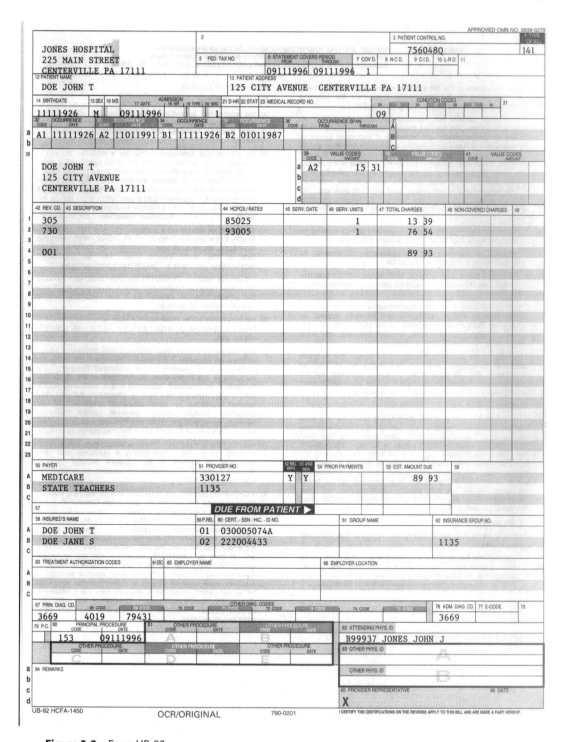

Figure 3-2 Form UB-92

Sample of EDI Claim Data

ASC X12N 837 INSTITUTIONAL HEALTH CARE CLAIM

Business Scenario—837 Institutional Claim

Patient is the same person as the Subscriber. The primary payer is Medicare and the secondary payer is State Teachers. The Bill is a 141 Type of Bill (Medicare patient coming to the hospital for referenced diagnostic services).

Primary Payer Subscriber: John T. Doe
Subscriber Address: 125 City Avenue, Centerville, PA 17111
Sex: M
DOB: 11/11/1926
Medicare insurance ID#: 030005074A
Payer ID #: 00435
Patient: Same as Primary Subscriber
Destination Payer: Medicare B
Submitter: Jones Hospital
EDI# 12345
Receiver: Medicare
EDI#: 00120
Billing Provider: Jones Hospital
Medicare Provider #330127
Address: 225 Main Street Barkley Building, Centerville, PA 17111
Attending Physician: John J. Jones
UPIN# B99937
Patient Account Number: 756048Q
Date of Admission: 09/11/1996
Statement Period Date: 09/11/1996–09/11/1996
Place of Service: Inpatient Hospital
Occurrence Codes and Dates:
     A1 11/11/1926
     A2 11/01/1991
     B1 11/11/1926
     B2 01/01/1987
Condition codes: 09
Value Codes: A2 $15.31
ICD-9 Procedure Codes and Dates: 15.3, 09/11/1996
Principal Diagnosis Code: 366.9
Secondary Diagnosis Codes: 401.9, 794.31
Number of Covered Days: 1
Services: Institutional Services Rendered:
Revenue Code: 305 HCPCS Procedure Code: 85025 Unit 1 Price $13.39
Revenue Code: 730 HCPCS Procedure Code: 93005 Unit 1 Price $76.54

Total Charges $89.93
Secondary Payer Subscriber: Jane S. Doe (wife)
Subscriber Address: 125 City Avenue, Centerville, PA 17111
Sex: M
DOB: 11/11/1926
State Teachers ID# 222004433
Payer ID #: 1135

Complete data string with each separate line as the computer writes it.
ST*837*987654~
BHT*0019*00*0123*19960918*0932*CH~
REF*87*004010X96~
NM1*40*2*MEDICARE*****46*00120~
PER*IC*JANE DOE*TE*9005555555~
NM1*41*2*JONES HOSPITAL*****46*12345~
HL*1**20*1~
PRV*BI*ZZ*203BA0200N~
NM1*85*2*JONES HOSPITAL*****XX*330127~
PRV*AT*ZZ*363LP0200N~
N3*225 MAIN STREET BARKLEY BUILDING~
N4*CENTERVILLE*PA*17111~
REF*G2*987654080~
HL*2*1*22*0~
SBR*P*18*******MB~
NM1*IL*1*DOE*JOHN*T***MI*030005074A~
N3*125 CITY AVENUE~
N4*CENTERVILLE*PA*17111~
DMG*D8*19261111*M~
NM1*PR*2*MEDICARE B*****PI*00435~
CLM*756048Q*89.93***14:A:1**Y*Y*Y~
DTP*434*D8*19960911~
CL1*3*1~
HI*BK:366.9~
HI*BF:401.9*BF:794.31~
HI*BQ:15.3:D8:19960911~
HI*BH:A1:D8:19261111*BH:A2:D8:19911101*BH:B1:D8:19261111*BH:B2:D8:198701
01~
HI*BE:A2:::15.31~
HI*BG:09~
NM1*71*1*JONES*JOHN*J***XX*B99937~
PRV*AT*ZZ*363LP0200N~
SBR*S*01*351630*STATE TEACHERS*GP****CI~
DMG***F~
OI***Y***Y~

```
NM1*IL*1*DOE*JANE*S***MI*222004433~
N3*125 CITY AVENUE~
N4*CENTERVILLE*PA*17111~
NM1*PR*2*STATE TEACHERS*****PI*1135~
LX*1~
SV2*305*HC:85025*13.39*UN*1~
DTP*472*D8*19960911~
LX*2~
SV2*730*HC:93005*76.54*UN*3~
DTP*472*D8*19960911~
SE*44*987654~
```

Each line begins with a computer code identifying the type of instruction. The end of each line finishes with a tilde (~). Looking through these lines of data you can find the Medicare ID number, the name and address of the service facility, and other information familiar to an insurance claim. Also listed are diagnosis codes, procedures, and their charges. Listed is the secondary insurance under Jane S. Doe with State Teachers insurance. The "header" lines are the first three beginning with ST, BHT and REF. These instructions begin the transaction and define the hierarchical type and the transmission type. At the end is the "trailer" instruction beginning with 'SE.' This informs the computer the transaction is over and to prepare to begin the next claim.

The next example is the data string as the computer records it. The data string is one long line transmitted without any spaces or line breaks. Once you know the ending markings and separators, you can begin to understand the information and correct errors when they occur. At the medical office the data string is not usually printed. This sample gives you an idea of just what is sent electronically and how the computer views the information.

ST*837*987654~BHT*0019*00*0123*19960918*0932*CH~REF*87*004010X96~NM1*40 *2*MEDICARE*****46*00120~PER*IC*JANE DOE*TE*9005555555~NM1*41 *2*JONES HOSPITAL*****46*12345~HL*1**20*1~PRV*BI*ZZ*203BA0200N~NM1*85*2*JONES HOSPITAL*****XX*330127~PRV*AT*ZZ*363LP0200N~N3*225 MAIN STREET BARKLEY BUILDING~N4*CENTERVILLE*PA* 17111~REF*G2 *987654080~HL*2* 1*22*0~SBR*P*18*******MB~NM1*IL*1*DOE*JOHN* T***MI*030005074A~N3*125 CITY AVENUE~N4*CENTERVILLE*PA*17111~DMG *D8*19261111*M~NM1*PR* 2*MEDICARE B*****PI*00435~CLM*756048Q* 89.93***14:A:1**Y*Y*Y~DTP*4 34*D8*19960911~CL1*3*1~ HI*BK:366.9~HI*BF:401.9*BF :794.31~HI*BQ:15.3:D8: 19960911~HI*BH:A1:D8:19261111*BH:A2:D8:19911101*BH:B1:D8:19261111*BH:B2:D8: 19870101~HI*BE:A2:::15.31~HI*BG:09~NM1*71*1*JONES*JOHN*J***XX*B99937~ PRV*AT*ZZ*363LP0200N~SBR*S*01*351630*STATE TEACHERS*GP****CI~DMG* **F~OI***Y***Y~NM1*IL*1*DOE*JANE*S***MI*222004433~N3*125 CITY AVENUE~N4*CENTERVILLE*PA*17111~NM1* PR*2*STATE TEACHERS *** **PI*1135~LX*1~SV2*305*HC:85025*13.39UN*1~DTP*472*D8*19960911~LX *2~SV2*730*HC:93005*76.54*UN3~DTP*472*D8*19960911~SE*44*987654~

LIMITATIONS TO CLAIMS ENCOUNTERS

Most insurance claims can be submitted electronically. However, there are still occasions when an attachment is necessary to fully explain the reasons for the charges listed. At this writing, the DHHS has not completed the adoption of a standard for attachments to claims/encounter transactions. In the future electronically transmitted claims with their attachments will be supported. The organization, Health Level Seven (HL7), is responsible to develop this standard. Until those standards are fully implemented, claims that require attachments will still be accepted on paper.

A limitation to an electronic health claim is the size of the file or loop iterations. The HIPAA ruling stipulates a limit of 99 service lines in a professional claim. This is sufficient for most claims. A health plan must be able to accept that number of lines when presented to them electronically. They cannot delay or deny processing a claim as long as it complies with the HIPAA Transaction Ruling.

REMITTANCE ADVICE AND SECONDARY PAYER

The original Health Care Claim X12N 837 form is information for each health plan that covers the patient. The *Health Care Claim Payment/Advice* ASC X12N 835-transaction returns information to the health care provider regarding payment and adjustments of payment. Some insurance claims are **crossover claims** going to more than one health plan. Each health plan and insured has their own set of benefits. Under HIPAA each plan must accept and process any transaction that meets the national standard. Each health plan listing the patient as a beneficiary will receive the same information and must process the claim in a timely manner. This allows for coordination of benefits with each responsible health plan. The transmission of the claim will not be returned to the provider until each health plan has had a chance to respond with their remittance advice. The health care provider is not to be penalized or the claim delayed when the payer receives claims for services they do not cover.

All claims must be processed no matter the content of the claim. Perhaps the charges included are not part of the coverage offered a particular patient. But perhaps the secondary payer or possibly the third payer does cover these charges. For example, prior to HIPAA, Medicare would accept claims for certain services and reject all others. Now Medicare must forego that policy and process all claims that meet HIPAA specifications. This does not mean that Medicare, or any other health plan, has to change payment policy. For instance, Medicare does not pay for a face-lift for cosmetic purposes only. With HIPAA standards implemented, Medicare is required to accept and process the bill, but still will not pay for a face-lift that is purely for cosmetic purposes (FAQs, 2003). Medicare will pass the claim electronically to the next payer for their review. Perhaps their benefits include payment at least in part for a face-lift for cosmetic purposes. The secondary or other payer will see the remittance advice from the primary payer and be able to make their determination about their reimbursement from the electronic information provided.

Prior to the HIPAA ruling, a provider would send a claim with information pertinent only to that first payer. After receiving the remittance advice, the health care provider would adjust the claim to include information for the secondary payer and a third payer if listed. Under HIPAA, the health care provider must include all information for all payers whether needed to adjudicate the health plan's claim or not. As stated in HIPAA law, each health plan receiving a standard transmission is not to delete any information given them even though it may not be important for the adjudication of their claim. That is administrative simplification in action.

Look at another example. One plan pays for a portion of home health services while another may not include that benefit. In compliance with HIPAA, the first payer must accept the transmission with all the home health data included. The payer cannot up-front reject such a claim. The payer is not required to bring that data into their adjudication system and provide payment. The payer, acting in accordance with policy and contractual agreements, can ignore data within the X12N 837 data set and pass the information on to the secondary payer.

WORKING WITH OUTSIDE ENTITIES

All health care providers need to have close communication with health plans that they transact business with electronically. The health plan and the health care provider are referred to as **Trading Partners**. Various types of trading partners are hospitals, physicians, health care payers, HMOs, PPOs, local, state, and federal governmental authorities, and trade organizations such as a hospital association. These entities may also be a Business Associate (BA) of the other entity. Health care providers may have a written Trading Partner Agreement with each of their trading partners. *This is not a requirement of HIPAA law.* It functions as protection between the health plan and health care provider so both parties understand the terms of partnership. If covered entities enter into a Trading Partner Agreement (TPA), the HIPAA rulings outline certain restrictions placed on such agreements.

Trading Partner Agreements

The agreement to conduct business electronically to transmit PHI is called a **Trading Partner Agreement (TPA).** This written document is an agreement related to the exchange of information in electronic transactions between each party. This definition allows for other arrangements to be formed between the two parties. TPAs may not modify the meaning of any values transmitted other than what is defined by the HIPAA Standards for Electronic Transactions. Both parties agree not to change any data element or segment to suit particular situations, nor to change the order in which segments are delivered between themselves. TPAs must also agree *not* to utilize any code or data in a manner that is unique to their communication. The HIPAA Officer is responsible for defining these agreements. When dependent on someone else for technical advice, the HIPAA Officer must make sure the vendor is doing reliable work on his behalf. It is the health care provider who is responsible to the CMS for compliance, not the software vendor. Payers are required by law to have the capability to send and receive all HIPAA transactions. Thus, it is imperative that trading partners be clear about specific data within the 837 transmissions they require or would prefer to have in order to efficiently adjudicate their claim (ASC X12N Guide, 2000).

Business Use and Definition

The ASC X12N standards minimize the need for users to reprogram their data processing systems for multiple formats. This is the driving force behind the Administrative Simplification portion of HIPAA. The transmission standards do not *define the method* in which interchange with trading partners is to take place. The link between hardware and translation software is flexible within the stated guidelines. The ASC success with other business and industry applications validates the simplicity of the open architecture format with wide variations in application. Each trading partner that will interface with another trading partner must meet HIPAA requirements individually.

SUMMARY

The HIPAA legislation mandates that when a health care provider and health plan communicate PHI electronically the transmission must comply with certain ASC X12N standards. In order to be sure that any health care provider has the resources to send claims to any health plan a uniform standard transaction was needed. The DHHS looked to industry standards endorsed by the ASC. The DHHS took the X12N transmissions designed by and for the insurance industry and added some file standards to fit the purposes of transmitting PHI. There are eight standard transactions that are endorsed by the DHHS that are to be used by health plans and health care providers as well as health care clearinghouses.

In order to standardize transactions, all parties must use the same *language* or code sets to communicate with each other. The medical code sets adopted are those that were generally in use prior to HIPAA law. The *ICD-9-CM* Volumes 1 and 2 is adopted to code diagnoses. Volume 3 of *ICD-9-CM* is designated to code inpatient procedures. Two standards are adopted to code physician and non-physician procedures for outpatients: CPT-4 and HCPCS. Dental procedures are to be coded from the *CDT-4* book. Each of these is updated regularly and only current codes are to be used. Non-medical codes needed to communicate other patient information in code form were adopted. They originated with the DHHS.

The transactions include claim forms; payment and remittance advice; inquiry and responses for eligibility; inquiry and response for determining the status of a particular claim; request for review to determine coverage and extent of reimbursement; and inquiry concerning enrollment status of a patient. The data sent electronically is in computer format yet is understandable by trained staff. Errors in data information can be found because the sequence of information is uniform and separators help locate invalid entries. Because all health plans receive claims electronically, this also allows for crossover claims to be transmitted electronically. Coordination of benefits is easier because all information is included in the first claim transmission.

Each health care provider and health plan has the option of TPAs. Trading Partners must abide by HIPAA rulings and not change any portion of electronic transmissions to suit their particular needs. The CMS, the designated enforcement agency for the DHHS, will look to the health care provider for compliance, not the software vendor. All HIPAA Officers need to be sure their office software is compliant since the responsibility rests with them.

END OF CHAPTER QUESTIONS

1. The Accredited Standards Committee develops and maintains standards for_____ for Electronic Data Interchange.

2. Certain health care providers are defined as those who _____ in electronic form.

3. Match the code with the type.

    A. *ICD-9-CM* Diagnosis (Diagnosis)

    B. *ICD-9-CM* Procedure (Inpatient procedure)

    C. *CPT-4* (Physician/outpatient procedure)

    D. HCPCS (Non-physician procedure)

    E. *CDT-4* (Dental procedures)

    1. _____ 052.9

    2. _____ 73.01

    3. _____ P9014

    4. _____ 76942

    5. _____ 93.94

    6. _____ 427.32

    7. _____ J3490

    8. _____ D7110

    9. _____ 99283

    10. _____ V70.3

    11. _____ 29125

    12. _____ 725.

    13. _____ 08.11

    14. _____ D1351

5. Two categories of code sets endorsed by HIPAA are _____ and _____ code sets.

6. The reference book to find the appropriate codes are:

    a. Diagnosis_____

    b. Physician procedures _____

    c. Hospital procedures _____

    d. Dental procedures _____

    e. HCPCS codes _____

7. Decide whether each of these is an example of Trading Partner (TP) or a Business Associate (BA) or both TP and BA:

    a. _____ A health care provider and software vendor

    b. _____ A health care provider and a health care clearinghouse

c. _____ A health care provider and a health plan

d. _____ A health care provider and a health insurance company

e. _____ A health care provider and a pharmacy

f. _____ A health care provider and the hospital where the physician practices

g. _____ A health care provider and an outside laboratory

h. _____ A health care provider and cleaning service for the office

8. The company that holds the copyright on Implementation Guides for HIPAA standard transactions is _____.

9. The Accredited Standards Committee set up templates for the transaction files. The structure is referred to as the _____ of the file.

10. Match the name of the transaction standard with the ID number assigned.

a. X12N _____ Health Care Services Review—Request and Response

b. X12N _____ Health Care Claim, Professional

c. X12N _____ Health Care Claim Status Request

d. X12N _____ Health Care Claim Payment/Advice

e. X12N _____ Health Care Claim, Institutional

f. X12N _____ Benefit Enrollment and Maintenance

g. X12N _____ Health Care Eligibility Benefit Inquiry

h. X12N _____ Health Care Claim Status Response

i. X12N _____ Health Care Claim, Dental

j. X12N _____ Health Care Eligibility Benefit Response

11. Transaction X12N 837 contains information about all health plans for the patient so that _____ ___ _____ with each health plan is automatic.

12. HIPAA ruling mandates that no health plan can reject a claim. What condition is placed on the health plan about information included in the standard transaction that is not important to adjudication?

Scenarios

How would you answer?

1. A state Medicaid plan enters into a contract with a managed care organization (MCO) to provide services to Medicaid recipients. That organization in turn contracts with different health care providers to render the services. When a health care provider submits a claim or encounter information electronically to the MCO, is this activity required to be a standard transaction?

2. In addition, the MCO then submits a bill to the state Medicaid agency for payment for all the care given to all the persons covered by that (MCO) for that month under a capitation agreement. Is this a standard transaction?

REFERENCES

ASC X12N Insurance Subcommittee Implementation Guide. (2000, May). A1 and 13.

Final Regulation Text: Standards for Electronic Transactions. (2000, July 25). Last modified Friday, January 31, 2003. Final Regulation Text: Standards for Electronic Transactions. Retrieved May 17, 2003 from http://www.cms.hhs.gov/hipaa/hipaa2/regulations/transactions/finalrule/txfin01.asp/

Frequently Asked Questions about Electronic Transactions Standards Adopted under HIPAA. (updated September 8, 2000). Retrieved September 8, 2003, from www.aspe.hhs.gov/admnsimp/ faqtx.htm p. 6.

Health Insurance Reform: Modifications to Electronic Data Transaction Standards and Code Sets, Final Rule. 68 Fed. Reg. 8,381–8,399 (February 20, 2003) (to codify 45 CFR Part 162).

Health Insurance Reform: Standards for Electronic Transactions, Final Rule. 65 Fed. Reg. 50,312–50,372. (August 17, 2000) (to codify 45 CFR Parts 160 and 162).

HIPAA Security Ruling

CHAPTER OUTLINE

Introduction

Core Requirements

  Administrative Safeguards

    Security Management

    Assigned Security Responsibility—
      Security Officer

    Workforce Security

    Information Access

    Security Awareness and Training

    Security Incidents

    Contingency Plan

    Evaluation of Security Effectiveness

    Business Associate Contracts

  Physical Safeguards

    Facility Access Controls

    Workstation Use or Access

    Workstation Security

    Device and Media Controls

  Technical Safeguards

    Access Control

    Audit Controls

    Integrity

    Person or Entity Authentication

    Transmission Security

  Organizational Requirements

  Policies, Procedures, and
    Documentation

Impact on Organizations

Challenges to Compliance

Summary

KEY TERMS

access	password
administrative safeguards	physical safeguards
algorithm	risk
audit trail	risk analysis
authentication	risk management
contingency plan	security of protected health information
encryption	security incident
information system	technical safeguards
infrastructure	user
integrity	workstation
nonrepudiation	

THINK ABOUT IT

1. Do privacy and security mean the same thing?

2. If a person's protected health information (PHI) is kept private, isn't it also secure?

True Story

About 400 pages of detailed psychological records concerning visits and diagnoses of at least 62 children and teenagers were accidentally posted on the University of Montana website for eight days. In most cases, the information included names, dates of birth and sometimes home addresses and schools attended with the results of the psychological tests.

—Piller, 2001

True Story

Confidential Medicaid records were disclosed during the sale of surplus equipment by the Arkansas Department of Human Services twice in six months. In October 2001, the state stopped the sale of the department's surplus computer storage drives when it was discovered that Medicaid records that were supposed to be erased were found on the computers. In April 2002, a man who bought a file cabinet from the department found the files of Medicaid clients in one of the cabinet's drawers. The files included four Social Security numbers and birth dates.

—DHS Surplus Sales, 2002

INTRODUCTION

The Security Rule is concerned with keeping protected health information (PHI) from unauthorized disclosures and safe from possible threats and hazards. This rule considers security different from privacy. To ensure privacy there must be a high level of security measures in place so unauthorized individuals do not gain access to information that is considered private. **Access** is considered the exposure necessary to read, write, modify, or communicate data and information. Access privilege is what allows an individual to enter a computer system for any purpose. The Internet transmission of electronic health claims must be protected from unauthorized access, loss, or modification. To keep electronic transmissions secure as defined in the Security Rule the covered entity must have hardware and software equipment that conforms to the **security** of PHI. Keeping PHI secure means there are safeguards (administrative, technical, or physical) in an information system that protect it and its information against unauthorized access, and limits access to authorized users in accordance with an established policy. Each covered entity must have the software programs that enable the information to be kept secure as well as available only to those authorized to access the information. Both of these requirements cost money and time to install and administer. The government has mandated five areas in which each covered entity must provide security for the PHI they process. These areas are (1) administrative safeguards, (2) physical safeguards, (3) technical safeguards, (4) organization requirements, and (5) policies, procedures, and documentation. Many of these concepts change the way business is conducted in the workplace. The Security Rule relies heavily on good technical support and expertise to keep the flow of information moving.

CORE REQUIREMENTS

The Department of Health and Human Services (DHHS) moved into the next phase of "accountability" in regard to PHI, that of ensuring the security of PHI that a covered entity maintains. Prior to HIPAA, paper copies of medical records were handled in a restricted manner to protect each patient's privacy. But little was done to provide backup copies in case of loss, disaster recovery, or for off-site storage. Certainly privacy and security are closely linked. Protecting the privacy of information depends largely on the existence of security measures to protect that information, yet security entails much more. The Privacy Rule sets standards for the disclosure and use of PHI. It restricts when, how, and how much health information can be provided if authorized. The new issue of security began with the move to electronic health information. There are many stories of computer hackers who access databases containing personal information of all kinds. The health care industry is particularly concerned about securing individually identifiable health information (IIHI). If appropriate care is not taken, information about the mental health status, HIV/AIDS condition, or general health status of an individual could end up in someone's possession without authorization. A disgruntled employee might misuse health information to discredit a co-worker. An estranged marriage partner, jealous or greedy family members, or business associates are other examples of individuals who can use protected health information dishonestly. By standardizing the requirement to secure health information, the DHHS believes every individual will be able to know that her personal health information is private *and* secure. There is a difference between keeping PHI private and keeping PHI secure. *All* PHI, no matter whether electronic, oral, paper, or film, must be protected and kept *private*. All PHI in *electronic* form must be kept *secure*. The focus of the Security Rule is on electronic information and the ways it is protected from invasion and accidental disclosure or loss.

Health information exists in many forms other than electronic data. Methods of transferring information such as paper-to-paper faxes, person-to-person telephone calls, video teleconferencing, and voice-mail messages are *not* subject to the Security Rule—even though they may contain electronic memory and can produce multiple copies. This list of excluded items also includes fax-back and voice response systems. A fax-back system is when a request for information is made via voice and the requested information is returned as a fax. The Security Rule does not apply in the previous illustration. The HIPAA Security Ruling covers *electronic* medical record systems and *electronic* order entry systems. That is, the data is stored in databases, text files, or any other binary format storage systems using computer storage media. The Security Rule also covers the binary *transmission* of data. Data at rest and data in transmission are affected, even if completely internal to a system.

All health care providers must be sure they comply with the Security Ruling in four core areas:

1. *Ensure confidentiality, integrity, and availability* of all electronic PHI they create, receive, maintain, or transmit.
2. *Protect against anticipated uses or disclosures* of any electronic information that is not permitted or required under the Privacy Rule.
3. *Protect against any anticipated threats or hazards* to the security, survivability, and integrity of PHI.
4. *Ensure compliance* with the Security Rule by their workforces (Ernst & Young, 2003).

Security requirements are organized into five categories: administrative safeguards, physical safeguards, technical safeguards, organizational requirements, and documentation. We will study each of these categories. In many ways privacy and security are interrelated. When covered entities work toward compliance with the Privacy Ruling, they must also comply with certain areas of the Security Ruling. But keeping PHI private does not necessarily mean it is fully secure. The DHHS covered many areas to be certain information is secure. Since this ruling includes small one-physician offices and large multi-campus teaching hospitals, the rules allow for interpretation to meet differing situations. However, every entity must meet certain standards while other requirements in the final plan can be adjusted. Some security issues are listed as required. Some issues are "addressable." The required items must be achieved and documented. Addressable items must be considered and solutions documented that are "reasonable and appropriate." When a health care provider finds a security issue that for them is not "reasonable and appropriate," the covered entity must document that decision of noncompliance and explain why it is not reasonable or appropriate for them. Documentation must include what the health care provider will substitute as an alternative policy or procedure in order to achieve the same goal. In all cases the covered entity must *document* what they are doing or not doing if they choose not to comply at this time. See Appendix B for a chart showing items that are required and those that are addressable.

Administrative Safeguards

The DHHS sets the standard but does not specify how to comply. The Security Rule mandates that each covered entity appoint someone to be responsible for securing electronic PHI. **Administrative safeguards** include administrative actions plus policies and procedures to manage the selection, development, implementation, and maintenance of security measures. The administrative safeguards also include managing the conduct of the covered entity's workforce in relation to the protection of PHI. During an audit the Centers for Medicare and Medicaid Services (CMS) will ask to see documentation that specifies how the entity is meeting the requirements of the Security Rule. These areas are:

- ❖ Security management
- ❖ Assigned security responsibility—security officer
- ❖ Workforce security
- ❖ Information access
- ❖ Security awareness and training
- ❖ Security incidents
- ❖ Contingency plans
- ❖ Evaluation of security effectiveness
- ❖ Business associate contracts

Security Management. The process of *security management* involves implementing policies and procedures to prevent, detect, and contain any intrusions of security. This is a required part of the Security Rule. The HIPAA Officer or designated Security Officer must conduct and maintain a risk analysis of the provider's organization. Before a health care provider can understand what they need to do to comply with the Security Rule they must find out where the threats are to electronic PHI. The administrator considers the cost of various security and control measures against the losses that would be expected if these measures were not in place. Each health care provider must look at the areas where PHI could be disclosed, lost, or modified in a way that is contrary to the Security Rule. The investigation must follow the path of electronic data and test each type of transmission or movement of data for any problems. The concept of **risk** is quite broad. It includes the impact and likelihood of an adverse event; the possibility of harm or loss to any software, information, hardware, administrative, physical, communications, or personnel resource within an automated information system or activity. That makes the administrator's responsibility to conduct a risk analysis a difficult task. The **risk analysis** focuses on the security of the computer system. The Security Officer must consider what cost-effective security and control measures may be selected to balance the cost of these security/control measures against the losses that would be expected if these measures were not in place. Once the risk analysis is completed, the covered entity is to write a plan to manage and minimize the risks they encountered. **Risk management** is the ongoing process that calculates the risk of the loss, disclosure, or modification of electronic information. Security measures are managed to offset threats and to keep the vulnerability of PHI to a minimal, acceptable level.

The risk analysis asks some important questions like:

- ❖ Who is able to view what information?
- ❖ Are there limits to the amount of information accessed by employees (i.e., a minimum necessary)?
- ❖ Is there an audit trail of who accessed or modified the record?
- ❖ Who can modify the information?
- ❖ How could this data be lost?
- ❖ What is the impact if the data cannot be recovered?

This investigation forms the basis for determining what areas need to be adjusted within the covered entity. The analysis must be documented for compliance. The study should indicate problems or gaps between current practices and what the Security Rule requires. Each health care provider must look at the measures they already have in place to provide security and reduce risks. Comparisons are then made with the additional measures needed to reach the level of compliance the Security Rule requires. An *adverse threat* is a transmission of PHI that is not secure with the result that information could be stolen, lost, or received by some party other than the intended entity. Any risks that are found must be documented. Once the risks are found, the next step is to decide how to manage those risks or to put new hardware, software, and policies in place to minimize the risk. The goal is to bring risks of disclosure or loss to a reasonable and bare minimum level. If the CMS requests a review of policy, the agents will expect to find a documented risk analysis as the first item completed and a written plan that was developed. The management portion of the security protections is meant to be scalable and flexible, so whether small or large, the covered entity can find a way to comply with the ruling. Cost considerations to bring the organization into compliance are also part of the decision-making process. These rulings are not funded—the government has not allowed for covered entities to receive payment for the mandated changes. Since each entity is to work toward compliance, the covered entity is expected to move in that direction and find a way they can pay for the changes.

Assigned Security Responsibility—Security Officer.   The administrator of each health care entity is to appoint a *Security Officer* whose responsibility is to develop and implement the policies and procedures required by the HIPAA Security Rule. This may be the same person as the Privacy Officer or HIPAA Officer mentioned in earlier chapters. The CMS looks to the Security Officer as the one responsible within the organization to administer and manage compliance. The officer takes the *risk analysis*—the difference between where the entity stands on compliance and where they need to be according to the Security Rule—and recommendations for change and sees to it that changes are made according to the written plan. The workforce must be trained in ways that ensure security measures are followed and limits to access are in place. The Security Officer is the one to oversee the management and supervision of persons in the workforce in relation to security issues. The Security Officer or other technology services person must regularly review audit logs and other security tracking reports. The Security Officer reviews who accessed electronic health information and when it was accessed. The Security Officer will need to periodically check for security threats or gaps as new equipment is purchased or software programs are updated. Another area for the Security Officer to check is Human Resource Department as employees leave the workforce or move from one department to another. Passwords and access to certain information need to be adjusted as employees change responsibilities. This standard is required.

Workforce Security. The responsibility for continued security within the workforce includes maintaining a record of access authorizations. One must ensure that operating and maintenance personnel have proper access authorization. After doing maintenance work, the maintenance access must be closed. Establishing personnel clearance procedures; establishing and maintaining security policies and procedures; and ensuring that system users have proper training are appropriate activities toward meeting the requirements. A **user** is a person with authorized access to the computer system. **Passwords** are a confidential numeric and/or character string used in conjunction with a User ID to verify the identity of the individual attempting to gain access to a computer system. Other things such as changing combination locks, removing a name from access lists, removing user account(s), and turning in of keys, tokens, or swipe cards that allow access are necessary to maintain the integrity of the security system. Maintaining the integrity of the system ensures data or information has not been altered or destroyed in an unauthorized manner. It may be necessary to change the authorization and delete or change passwords to prevent unauthorized access to electronic information. This standard is addressable. Each entity determines what fits. Some providers have implemented biotechnology for security. A small provider may find this too expensive. There is no one solution to security issues. All procedures are to be documented and in that manner the entity is considered in compliance.

Information Access. Each covered entity must have in place policies for implementing and maintaining the appropriate level of access for all personnel authorized to view health information. This standard is required. Each job description carries with it the explanation of the extent of information needed to perform that job adequately. Access should be limited to the minimum necessary as stated in the Privacy Rule. The access should not restrict anyone from completing her job responsibilities relating to health care, billing, or normal operations.

Security Awareness and Training. Training is important for all workforce employees, for physicians, and for volunteers. Training should also include administration personnel because they have access to electronic information. The training stimulates awareness about the vulnerability of data within the electronic system and the ways to ensure its safety. The workforce ought to know about virus protection measures. Training should include how to immediately report any event that might mean the protection has been compromised. Proper login and logoff procedures lessen the possibility of unauthorized access to health information. Training should include appropriate password usage and proper changes of passwords to ensure the safety of the system. Since each health care provider is different, this standard is addressable. Each Security Officer is to meet the standard for training and awareness as it best fits her organization.

Security Incidents. A **security incident** is defined as the attempted or successful unauthorized access, use, disclosure, modification, destruction of information, or interference with system operations in an **information system**. An information system normally includes hardware, software, information, data, applications, communications, and people. It interconnects information resources under the same direct management control that share a common functionality or purpose. The DHHS defines this attempted or successful unauthorized access into an information system a security incident rather than a security breach. PHI may not have been compromised but the possibility exists—hence, the use of the word incident. This is a required standard. In response to an incident, the HIPAA Security Rule mandates that there be a formal, documented response and report written and executed. All authorized workers are expected to report a security incident no matter what the size or origin. The health care provider is better off taking steps early to protect information and prevent a larger problem. This minimizes exposure and will keep PHI from being shared or accessed. Sometimes the incident will involve another covered entity. Advising a covered entity immediately that a security incident has occurred is part of expected business practice. This will help the other entity to contain the possible breach of security at their end and advise them of the need to report the incident too.

Contingency Plan. Many people are frightened of the notion of disaster plans and contingency planning. They perceive these to be very costly and difficult to manage. Something that *may* happen but is not likely to happen is hard to imagine. A **contingency plan** for security consists of having policies and procedures in place to respond to an emergency or other occurrence that damages systems containing electronic PHI. The reality of a disaster, whether local or more widespread, is a possibility that requires planning. No locality is immune from natural disasters. No one can guarantee complete protection against a terrorist attack or from human error. If disaster strikes, can individuals get access to their health information? Can information be accessed from an offsite location? Each covered entity must have a plan in place and maintain that plan even as equipment and staff change.

Because there is no guarantee regarding emergencies, it is required that a contingency plan be in place. Items in this plan include:

- ❖ Applications and data critical analysis
- ❖ A data backup plan
- ❖ A disaster recovery plan
- ❖ An emergency mode operation plan
- ❖ Testing and revision procedures

Covered entities must consider how any disaster could damage systems that contain electronic PHI and develop policies and procedures for responding to such situations. Having backup data stored offsite and recycled on a regular basis is part of a contingency plan. Consideration should be given to how business can continue if it is not possible to continue working in the present facility. What measures need to be taken to begin again in a new location?

Evaluation of Security Effectiveness. The HIPAA Security Rule requires that each covered entity periodically conduct an evaluation of their security safeguards. This periodic check will document the compliance with HIPAA ruling on a routine basis. Any time there is new equipment brought on line, new software installed or updated, or facility changes, they should be evaluated as to their effectiveness and compliance with HIPAA. In this way, documentation of compliance will be current and ready when needed.

Business Associate Contracts. Part of the Business Associate (BA) contract written under the Privacy Rule involves satisfactory assurance that the BA will appropriately safeguard PHI it receives and/or transmits. The Security Officer must review all contracts with BAs. All covered entities have agreements to deal with the Privacy Ruling. An appendix (addition) may be necessary to add wording to cover the Security Rule regulations. The contract between the covered entity and the BA must include provisions that the BA will:

❖ Implement safeguards that are reasonable and appropriate to protect the confidentiality, integrity, and availability of electronic PHI it creates, receives, maintains, or transmits.
❖ Ensure that any agent (staff member) who may be entrusted with such information agrees to the same safeguards.
❖ Report to the covered entity *any* security incident of which it becomes aware.
❖ Authorize termination of the contract if the covered entity determines that the BA has violated the contract.

Physical Safeguards

The next focus of security deals with equipment and the physical storage and maintenance of PHI. The **physical safeguards** include physical measures, policies, and procedures to protect a covered entity's electronic information systems and related equipment from all hazards and from unauthorized intrusions. The items required under physical safeguards for security cover four areas. They are:

1. Facility access controls: buildings, computers, and server rooms
2. Workstation use or access
3. Workstation (software) security
4. Device and media controls

Facility Access Controls. Facility access deals with gaining entry to areas where PHI is stored as well as access to the physical location where computer hardware is located. The Security Officer must document how her particular organization is addressing physical access—the specifics are considered addressable. The specifics must include:

❖ Disaster recovery
❖ Emergency mode operation
❖ A facility security plan
❖ Procedures for verifying access authorizations before any access is permitted

Physical access to computer information system hardware is limited to only those workers who need to administer and maintain the electronic systems where PHI is stored. Limiting access involves keeping doors locked and requiring the use of keys or electronic locks. An advantage of electronic locks is their capability to record the time of entry and who entered. Other items that need to be considered are the maintenance records, need-to-know procedures for personnel access, and sign-in/sign-out records for visitors and visitor escorts. A typical checklist to meet HIPAA Physical Security includes questions like:

❖ How do you access the building?
❖ Are closed circuit cameras recording?
❖ Is there an employee entrance?
❖ Are the doors manual or electric?
❖ Can access be gained from the loading dock or garage?
❖ How do visitors gain access to the building?
❖ Are business visitors escorted at all times?

This last question considers business visitors other than patients and their visitors. It refers to business visitors who may enter parts of the building where they would have access to equipment that holds and maintains PHI.

Some questions dealing with health information in the *patient care areas*:

❖ Are medical records stored securely?
❖ Are they protected from fire, loss, theft, etc.?
❖ Can PHI be easily viewed?

The Security Officer must continuously provide reasonable safeguards for each of these situations and document them in the policy manual for security.

Workstation Use or Access. The definition of **workstation** is an electronic computing device, for example, a laptop or desktop computer, a personal data assistant (PDA), or any other device that performs similar functions, and has electronic media stored in its immediate environment. No matter where these are located inside a facility, workstation access to information is to be limited to the job description. A workstation "logoff" procedure is very important to minimize unauthorized access to health information. Auto logoff is a requirement. Time delay is not specified, but a 10-minute delay to logoff is a good maximum for most situations, even in "secure" areas.

Workstation (Software) Security. Each person on the workforce should understand the Internet use policy as well as the email policy of the entity. Equipment at work is to be used only for business—not personal use. Training should include how to save computer files for backup security and how to transmit PHI when needed. Some questions dealing with workstation security are:

❖ Does the workforce understand how to lock their computer screen?
❖ Are passwords, tokens, or biometrics used to secure workstations?
❖ Can workstation screens be viewed by passers-by?
❖ Are encryption processes in place where needed?

Security standards extend to members of a provider's workforce whether they work on site or at home. Any transcriptionists or other workers who have been authorized to work from their home must have the same security protections as those employees working on site. "At home" workers are defined as part of a covered entity's workforce and are a special high risk. Information systems personnel must extend security to all off-site locations. Any security incidents must be reported immediately and procedures implemented to remedy the situation. These off-site locations must be protected and monitored as closely as on-site workstations.

Device and Media Controls. The Security Officer must keep a record of the receipt and removal of all central processing unit (CPU) hardware and clinical software that is used within the facility. This provides a means to track when hardware items are purchased. When that item is considered obsolete, the Security Officer must have a record of its disposition. Disks, tapes, hand-held devices, cell phones, and similar electronic communication devices are also items that are covered by this portion of the ruling. Electronic devices can hold many types of PHI. The Security Rule requires that disposal and reuse of equipment and media be documented. This rule covers disposal of *all* forms of media that contains PHI. The information may be on backup tapes and disks, or other data storage media. It can also be on thermal transfer ribbons from fax machines and label printers. The Security Officer needs to compile an inventory of all equipment containing PHI. The list must contain the date when it entered the system and when it was disposed, how it was disposed, and measures taken to destroy any unneeded information that is protected. Just how the officer meets these standards is an addressable issue since each organization varies. These devices must be erased, deleted, or destroyed in an appropriate manner when discarded. This prevents them from being resold or recycled to the public who unknowingly receive information that should have been deleted, destroyed, or erased. The following true story illustrates problems addressed by the Security Officer.

True Story

A Nevada woman who purchased a used computer discovered that the computer still contained the prescription records of the customers of the pharmacy that had previously owned the computer. The pharmacy database included names, addresses, social security numbers, and a list of all the medicines the customers had purchased.

—Markoff, 1997

Technical Safeguards

Technical safeguards mean the technology and the policy and procedures that protect electronic PHI at rest or in transmission. There are several items relating to the **infrastructure** that need to be in place to ensure the security of electronic PHI. The infrastructure is the wiring or basic network of a system or organization. Here infrastructure means the computer server(s), the hubs, switches, connecting wires, terminals or workstation PCs, and the rooms or closets where they are located (Briggs, 2004). These must be kept secure from intrusion.

The Security Officer must address issues dealing with:

1. Access control
2. Audit controls

3. Integrity (of electronic PHI)
4. Person or entity authentication
5. Transmission security

The DHHS includes a certification standard for technical systems and software that each covered entity must meet in order to be in compliance. The Department does not define *how* to meet the requirements.

Access Control. Access control prevents unauthorized people (or unauthorized processes) from entering the information technology system. This is an addressable item for compliance. Several methods regulate access control: a personal identification number (PIN), a password system, or a biometric identification system. Biometric identification uses a part of the body to authenticate the individual such as the iris of the eye, fingerprint shape recognition, or handprint. A telephone callback or token system can be used to verify the user. Robust firewalls and anti-virus protection must be in place. There needs to be a method of electronically blocking unauthorized external access to local area networks (LANs). One requirement of access control is to install automatic logoff at workstations. The method for securing workstations is not specified so entities can find the best fit to their particular situation. Some of the questions the Security Officer must address are:

❖ Is the list of approved authorized users maintained and updated regularly?
❖ Are unauthorized intrusion efforts adequately blocked?
❖ Are personnel files matched with user accounts to be sure workers who have been terminated or transferred do not retain unnecessary system access?
❖ Are passwords changed every 90 days or sooner and not easily guessed?
❖ Are passwords hidden when entered?
❖ Are passwords stored securely and according to the policy?
❖ Are temporary vendor passwords deleted immediately?
❖ Does the workstation limit the number of invalid access attempts that may occur for a given user?
❖ Are robust anti-virus measures in place?

Passwords should not be easily guessed. They should be a minimum of seven characters with a mix of upper and lower case letters and numbers. It currently takes a hacker less than a minute to guess any combination of four characters. With current computer speeds, a hacker will take several hours to guess a five-character code and several weeks to guess a seven-character code. Good security demands proper usage of passwords and a regular schedule to change them. An industry standard for any business organization mandates a change of passwords every 90 days or sooner. The expectation for the Security Rule is no different.

HIPAA does not require the use of electronic signatures, but there is a movement within the industry toward maintaining totally electronic medical records. This eliminates additional paper being added to the medical record but adds the problem of keeping electronic health information secure. Electronic signatures will be necessary if a health care provider chooses to move to a paperless environment. Electronic signatures must provide the combination of authenticity, message integrity, and "nonrepudiation" that is necessary in an electronic environment. **Nonrepudiation** means a method by which the sender of data is provided with proof of delivery and the recipient is assured of the sender's identity, so that neither can later deny having processed the data. Some signatures reproduce the actual written signature as an image and place that on the document through password protection. Other systems require a set of passwords and then print the physician's name, date, the time, and the statement "This is electronically signed" to the document. To date, the DHHS has not adopted a standard for electronic signatures. This technology is still evolving. The government is sure that viable solutions will be available soon. Until that time, the electronic signature requirements in the HIPAA ruling are not addressed.

Audit Controls. The security standards emphasize the need to train persons about the value of **audit trails** in computerized record systems. An audit trial examines the information system activity to track which password or station accessed information (who: login ID); what information was accessed and what was done to it (read-only, modify, delete, add, etc.); and when (date/timestamp). Changes to the information are allowed for a limited time. After a specified time, the information entered into the electronic system must be permanent. Only addendums are then permitted. This way there is a record of the original entry, the adjustments to it, and the timing of the change. Some questions to answer are:

- ❖ Does the audit trail support "after-the-fact" investigations of how, when, and why normal operations ceased?
- ❖ Is access to online audit logs strictly controlled?
- ❖ Is there a separate person in charge of administering access control functions from the person who administers the audit trail?
- ❖ Is suspicious activity investigated and appropriate action taken?

Integrity. The definition of **integrity** of PHI means that the entity is required to confirm that data in its possession is accurate and has not been altered, lost, or destroyed in an unauthorized manner. This section of the Security Rule looks at protecting data from accidental or malicious alteration and destruction. It is designed to provide assurance to the user that the information meets federal expectations about its quality and integrity. The Security Officer must consider issues such as:

- ❖ Is virus detection and virus elimination software installed and activated?
- ❖ Is any inappropriate or unusual activity reported and investigated, and appropriate action taken?
- ❖ Are intrusion detection tools installed on the system?

Clearly many of these items require sophisticated knowledge of information systems and their functions. For this reason, this standard is addressable to meet the needs of the health care provider.

Person or Entity Authorization. Anyone logging on to the electronic system must be identified by some method, usually a user ID or password. Care must be taken to keep passwords private and changed on a regular basis. Authorization systems must limit the times a user can attempt access if the attempt is not accurate. Authentication or the confirmation that a person is the one claimed must be secure and updated as employees move or change responsibilities. With electronic claims submission, the computer system must be able to identify the entity that is sending the information as well as who is receiving it.

Transmission Security. The Security Rule requires protection of transmitted PHI. The data must be protected in a manner corresponding to the associated risk. This may mean using **encryption** technology as the data is sent over the Internet or dial-up lines. Encryption technology changes readable text into a vast series of "garbled" characters using complex mathematical **algorithms** (a step-by-step procedure for solving a problem). Another way of defining encryption is using an algorithmic process to transform data into a format in which there is a low probability of assigning meaning to the result without using a confidential process or key. Once encrypted, data can be transmitted over unsecured lines. Because older codes can be easily broken, the encryption technology needs to be re-evaluated routinely. With the introduction of wireless devices, like hand-held devices, tablet PCs, and notebooks, security through encryption is difficult to achieve. Many software companies are working to improve this technology to bring security and integrity of data to wireless devices. Point-to-point communication via modem is considered to be secure. A virtual private network (VPN) is a point-to-point "tunnel" through the Internet accomplished by a special encryption technique. Encryption is left as an addressable issue. The specifics of encryption are up to the covered entity.

Organizational Requirements

The organization requirements focus mainly on the aspect of BA contracts. This section also covers certain requirements that health plans must meet. Covered entities are required to have appropriate contracts with all BAs. Within the contract with all BAs are provisions stating that all reasonable and appropriate safeguards must be in place. The BA is to protect the confidentiality, integrity, and availability of the electronic form of PHI that they create, receive, maintain, or transmit. Part of the organization requirements is that any security incident must be documented and reported to the other entity. If violations are found with a particular BA, and reasonable and appropriate safeguards have not been in place, then the covered entity is to terminate the contract with that BA.

Health care clearinghouses process a large portion of the total volume of health claims. They provide a service to providers by filtering claims from many health care providers through their editing system to ensure accuracy. They adjust claims to fit the needs of the various health plans. The clearinghouse then forwards the claims in large batches to the specific health plans. They act as an intermediary. Each provider does not have to be concerned with the specifics of health plan requirements. These clearinghouses must maintain security of all PHI they process just as a health care provider must. The same measures implemented by a health care provider or health plan are to be used and documented by health care clearinghouses. The BA contract between the clearinghouse and the health care provider must state that reasonable and appropriate safeguards are in place to protect the confidentiality, integrity, and availability of the electronic PHI they process.

Policies, Procedures, and Documentation

The Security Rule requires that all policies be accessible for review either in electronic form or on paper in a manner that is readily available to all employees. These policies should be reviewed on a regular basis to ensure compliance. They must be updated regularly as rulings change. The Security Officer is to consult the DHHS regularly to determine if changes have been posted that affect the health care provider. All documentation of policies and procedures are to be kept for six years even though the wording has changed or been eliminated. This allows an investigator to go back to what a policy said six years ago even though the current policy may read differently. This means if an incident is under investigation, documentation is still available to see what steps were in force at the time of the incident.

IMPACT ON ORGANIZATIONS

Physicians' offices and clinics face the challenge to continue business without interruption to patients while changing procedures to comply with HIPAA. Where the physician practice is small, the burden of compliance falls on a very limited number of workers. Entities may not have money available to readily purchase equipment and technical assistance to comply in a short time. The DHHS sees this change to HIPAA compliance as a pathway. The DHHS is encouraging covered entities to begin moving toward compliance in small steps. As long as an investigator is able to find willingness to change and movement toward complying with the Security Rule, enforcement agents will encourage compliance rather than issue penalties. The Office of HIPAA Standards is a division of the DHHS. This office is responsible for enforcement of the Security Rule. The deadline for compliance with the Security Rule is April 20, 2005, for health plans, health care clearinghouses, and health care providers. However, if the health plan qualifies as a small health plan, providers have another year to be compliant—until April 20, 2006. There is no penalty for initiating these standards prior to the deadline. For those in the medical office, electronic health claims to small health plans may not yet be standardized and secure as defined by Security Ruling until April 2006.

Many hospitals encounter budget shortfalls. There are often cutbacks in federal reimbursements. Private health plans have also revised their payments and lowered reimbursements. Insurance coverage of prescriptions has had to balance the increasing usage of medications and their increasing cost against maintaining premiums that individuals can afford. It is hard for many hospitals to provide funds to cover the initial cost of the standards. The DHHS has purposely written the standards to be "technology neutral." No one product has all the answers to security requirements. Yet the challenge is to build a technology base and infrastructure that will be able to grow and meet the requirements.

A technology that is increasingly utilized is telemedicine. Telemedicine uses videoconferencing to conduct an office visit with a physician located at a distant location. Many hospitals, both large and small, are becoming involved with this means of conducting patient encounters. This is referred to as an *interactive videoconferencing consultation*. Using the Internet a patient can have an office visit with a physician located many miles away. The patient is monitored locally and the health information and visual images are transmitted to the consulting physician. The consulting physician can watch the patient move, walk, or perform other activities just as if she were in the room. Generally, a physician's assistant is on site to conduct any tests or procedures the consulting doctor may request. The discussion between patient and physician via videoconferencing bring both parties together so well that the idea of distance is forgotten. It may seem as if the doctor and patient are actually in the same location. Often these office visits/consultations are videotaped so either the consulting physician or local provider can review the interview and provide a report.

The DHHS has submitted the following definition for security of these videotapes. The videotapes themselves are not part of the medical record and should be erased after standard documentation of care is complete. The patient must provide written consent before the taping begins. Written consent may be omitted if the documentation relates to abuse or neglect. Under usual circumstances, the videotape would be erased shortly after the encounter and the only record of the teleconference would be the electronic or paper report with the physician's signature. The physician's report is to include the final disposition of the videotape: whether it was erased, not erased, and where it will be kept (Telehealth Update, 2000). Tapes may be kept that have educational value to medical students. If any educational tapes are retained, they must not have any personal identifiers. They must be de-identified as specified under the Privacy Ruling of HIPAA. There is no requirement to tape the sessions. An unrecorded telemedicine video transmission is not yet considered PHI.

CHALLENGES TO COMPLIANCE

The DHHS has written Security Rules in a manner that applies to any organization, regardless of size. The challenge is to enhance efficiency in the process of paying the provider for health care, and at the same time reduce the costs involved with doing business. Many entities will experience initial cost involved in changing hardware and/or software systems. As implementation continues, the return on the investment will grow. This will happen through simplifying the administration of claims. The time needed to prepare health claims for submission will also decrease.

The federal government understands that it is impossible to keep PHI totally secure. The goal of the DHHS is to encourage documentation that the covered entity, whether a health care provider, health care clearinghouse, or health plan, has taken steps to ensure the safety and security of PHI. This means a balance must be made between the identifiable risks and the cost of protective measures. As with the Privacy Rule, the rule of thumb is to provide reasonable and appropriate security for the particular situation the covered entity encounters. The risk analysis and risk management plans are basic to compliance. These risk documents are part of the documentation maintained by the Security Officer. The challenge in managing the security process comes in identifying the necessary changes in addition to finding the people and resources qualified to bring about the required changes.

A typical hospital workforce includes both paid and non-employee workers (physicians), making enforcement of security standards more challenging. Many hospitals utilize a large number of volunteer workers to perform routine hospital responsibilities. Including volunteer workers in the workforce adds another challenge to security management.

Day-to-day access to the health care facility must be protected. At the same time, visitors and those with physical handicaps should not be hindered from gaining entrance and exit. Doors need to be monitored to reduce the risk of theft or unintended disclosure of information. The Security Officer needs to balance the risk of a particular situation with the cost of preventing unauthorized access to health information.

A big challenge in keeping transmissions secure is the increasing use of Internet communication. Most Internet-based email is not sent in an encrypted format. PHI cannot be emailed unless a security algorithm is in place. More and better wireless technology is available and requires special attention to keep information secure.

SUMMARY

The HIPAA Security Rule covers any PHI that is in electronic form. This may be information that is transmitted or "at rest"—stored at a health care provider's facility. The Privacy Rule protects health information from being used or disclosed in ways that are not authorized either for means of treatment, payment, or normal health care business operations. The Security Rule expects that health information be kept protected. Procedures must be in place to maintain the integrity of the data within information systems. Access to necessary information is to be available only to those authorized to view the health information. Security includes protection against anticipated threats or hazards. In order to comply with the federal ruling, each covered entity must consider five main areas of compliance: administrative safeguards, physical safeguards, technical safeguards, organization requirements, and policy and procedure documentation.

The administration of each entity must analyze the risks within their organization utilizing a *risk analysis*. They must then develop a plan to minimize the risks of unauthorized disclosure or access to the electronic health information they maintain with a *risk management* plan. One specific person is to be the *Security Officer*. This officer may oversee a security committee depending upon the size of the entity. Each person on the workforce must be trained in the use of security measures to access the information needed to perform his or her job. The information access is limited to the "minimum necessary" as explained in the Privacy Rule. If any attempted or successful security incident is found, the incident is to be documented and steps taken to remedy the situation immediately. Each covered entity must have written *contingency plans* in place for disasters of any kind. The Security Rule expects periodic evaluations of the safeguards to measure their effectiveness. All BA contracts must have additional information to safeguard PHI the associate may encounter in the course of doing business.

The physical security of the building, electronic storage equipment, and workstations is the focus of the second portion of the Security Rule. *Access* to locations where protected health information is stored must be secure. All *workstations* must be located to maximize security and software logoff timers must be in place to minimize unauthorized access. Any electronic device, whether stationary or portable, that contains PHI must be logged, especially when it is taken out of service. The Security Officer is expected to oversee that information held within these devices is erased, deleted, or destroyed appropriately.

Within the management of electronic equipment, there must be controls of the levels of access dependent upon the job description. An *audit trail* must be present to trace data movement and access. *Authentication* must be secure and updated as employees move or change responsibilities. Under the technical safeguards, the transmission of protected health information must be kept secure through *encryption* methods.

As of 2003 there were an estimated 4 million health plans and another 1.2 million health care providers in addition to many health care clearinghouses that facilitated the claims between providers and payers. All of these entities will consider moving to an electronic information system because the cost of continuing with paper forms is much more costly than the cost of storing and transmitting health information electronically. If the cost of change is currently too great, either the health plan or health care provider may continue with paper copies of PHI. The Security Ruling of HIPAA will not apply to the covered entity if that is their choice. However, if *any* of their information is kept or transmitted in electronic format, then the Security Rule must be adopted, with appropriate policies and procedures implemented to ensure compliance.

END OF CHAPTER QUESTIONS

1. A covered entity must comply with the Security Rule if _____ protected health information (PHI) is kept or transmitted.

2. Give three examples of information not covered by the Security Rule.

   _____

3. The Security Rule covers only the _____ _____ of health information.

4. The _____ _____ is the person who is responsible to _____ and _____ policies and procedures required by HIPAA.

5. The Security Officer is responsible to see that the _____ _____ is conducted and all risks and gaps are addressed to minimize possible disclosures.

6. Information available to each employee is to be the _____ _____ to perform their job effectively.

7. Training of staff members includes categories such as _____, _____, _____, and _____.

8. Can one physician's office FAX patient medical information to another physician's office? Is this considered a confidential means of communication?

9. True/False—HIPAA specifies how often security effectiveness is to be evaluated.

10. True/False—People employed to work at home are considered Business Associates.

11. True/False—Computer closets/rooms must be kept locked in order to comply with the Security Rule.

12. True/False—Tapes made during a videoconference consultation are to be stored as part of the medical record.

13. The Security Officer must have inventory of all electronic equipment that is _____ from the facility to ensure no PHI is included.

14. Health care clearinghouses help health care providers and health plans by acting as _____ between providers and payers.

15. Any policy that is written to show compliance with the Security Rule must be kept on file for _____ years.

16. Match the terms with their definitions:

Security incident _____

Risk analysis _____

Contingency plan _____

Clearinghouse _____

    A. A process whereby cost-effective security and control measures may be selected by balancing the cost of various security/control measures against the losses that would be expected if these measures were not in place

    B. A plan including applications and data criticality analysis, a data backup plan, a disaster recovery plan, an emergency mode operation plan, and testing and revision procedures

    C. The attempted or successful unauthorized access, use, disclosure, modification, destruction of information, or interference with system operations in an information system

    D. Receives a standard transaction from another entity and processes or facilitates the processing of information into nonstandard format or nonstandard data content for a receiving entity

Scenarios

How would you answer?

1. A hacker downloaded medical records, health information, and social security numbers on more than 5,000 patients at the University of Washington Medical Center. The hacker was motivated by a desire to expose the vulnerability of electronic medical records (O'Harrow, 2000).

    a. What protections should be in place to protect from this kind of theft?
    b. How do HIPAA security rules create an environment that prevents this from happening again?

2. A physician was diagnosed with AIDS at the hospital in which he practiced medicine. His surgical privileges were suspended (Estate of Behringer v. Medical Center at Princeton, 1991).

a. Were his privacy rights under HIPAA violated through this security breach?

b. Does knowing this type of information violate the staff member's privacy?

Scenario of a patient encountering HIPAA during a hospital visit.

Concepts identified in Scenario that are HIPAA-related:

access to psychotherapy notes

audit trail

authenticated

authorization requirements

Business Associate

business as usual

cases of victims of abuse, neglect, or domestic violence

Covered Entity

data backup and disaster recovery plan

definition of health care operations

de-identified

designated ANSI X12 standard format

designated code sets

designated record set

disclosure of protected health information

encrypted

hospital directory

individually identifiable health information (IIHI)

identifier standards

minimum necessary

need to know

non-repudiation security

normal operations

Notice of Privacy Practices

"opt-out" of future requests

personal representatives

protected health information (PHI)

purposes/reasons of treatment, payment, or health care operation (TPO)

release of directory information

request to amend

research study

standardized transmission request/reply

training

unauthorized access

victim(s) of abuse, neglect, or domestic violence

written accounting of disclosures

Scenario: HIPAA Rules in Practice

1. The mayor's elderly mother, Mrs. Elsa Goodman, is found unconscious at her home by a neighbor. The neighbor calls for an ambulance. The Emergency Department (ED) doctor on duty, Dr. Eveready, begins resuscitation; finds a broken arm, badly bruised chest, and other bruises on her body. Registration clerk begins to enter patient information into the hospital system.

    a) The registration clerk needs to be trained in privacy and security matters. The hospital must document this *training.*

    b) The system should maintain an *audit trail* of information viewed and modified showing who did what and when.

    c) The registration clerk needs to have been *authenticated* by the system, and his authority to perform the registration task confirmed.

2. Mrs. Goodman's primary care physician (PCP), Dr. Karing, is on the medical staff at the hospital. The Emergency Department gains access to Mrs. Goodman's records and prints out progress notes from her last office visit.

    a) The printer must be protected from *unauthorized access*.

    b) The progress notes are *protected health information* (PHI). All *individually identifiable health information (IIHI)* created, stored, or transmitted in either electronic or paper formats are specifically protected under HIPAA.

    c) The security rule requires an *audit trail showing who accessed the record and for what purpose.* Although the rule does not specify *the mechanics* of the audit trail, it is prudent to have a tracking mechanism for paper printouts and assign responsibility for monitoring their use and disposition.

    d) The Transaction and Code Set Rule require a *data backup and disaster recovery plan*.

3. A notation from Primary Care Physician, Dr. Karing, shows that Mrs. Goodman had seen a psychotherapist for depression. Dr. Eveready requests the psychotherapist's notes to determine possible overdose of medications.

    a) HIPAA has special *authorization requirements* for *access to psychotherapy notes*. The general consent requirement for use and disclosure of PHI for treatment, payment, and health care operations *does not extend* to psychotherapy notes. However, HIPAA allows for emergency access in those circumstances where the patient is unresponsive.

b) A **Business Associate** Agreement between Dr. Eveready and the psychotherapy facility is not required, because Dr. Eveready is a provider who will use the information for treatment of Mrs. Goodman.

c) The psychotherapy facility must **authenticate** Dr. Eveready. The **minimum necessary** standard does not apply, because Dr. Eveready is a health care provider requesting information to be used in treating Mrs. Goodman.

 i) Included in psychotherapy notes are:

 (l) Notes recorded by a mental health professional documenting or analyzing the contents of a conversation during a private, group, joint, or family counseling session.

 (2) Psychotherapy notes are filed separately from the rest of the individual's medical record.

 ii) Excluded from psychotherapy notes are

 (1) Medication prescriptions

 (2) Modalities and frequency of treatment

 (3) Results of clinical tests and summaries of diagnoses

 (4) Functional status

 (5) Treatment plans

 (6) Symptoms, prognosis, and progress

4. The Emergency Department sees a prescription for medicine that could be a possible suicide drug. The Emergency Department requests STAT report but the local hospital lab does not perform this test—it is sent to an outside lab.

a) The reference lab does not have to provide a **notice of its privacy practices** to Mrs. Goodman even though they are a provider of services because it is an indirect provider.

b) A **Business Associate** contract is not required for the reference lab because it is an indirect health care provider, and this is a normal health care operation.

5. The Primary Care Physician's file that was accessed by the registration clerk indicates that the mayor, Mr. Goodman, has power of attorney for health care. Mr. Goodman is notified of his mother's condition.

a) Disclosure of protected health information is permitted to those who have been given authority to "stand in the shoes," **personal representatives**, of the patient to exercise the patient's rights.

6. Ambulance personnel notify local authorities of their suspicion of elderly abuse from information gained from the neighbor who called them, as well as viewing the unhealthy living conditions they found in Mrs. Goodman's home.

   a) Information may be disclosed without Mrs. Goodman's authorization or Mr. Goodman's authorization if there is reason to believe the patient has been a ***victim of abuse, neglect, or domestic violence.***

7. The patient's clinical information is entered into the hospital computer system by the Emergency Department staff and is displayed on a monitor in the Emergency Department's patient room.

   a) Patient information is not to be available to anyone other than those involved in the treatment of the patient. The monitors cannot display ***protected health information*** so that other patients, family members, or employees and staff without proper authority or the ***"need to know"*** can view it.

8. Mrs. Elsa Goodman regains consciousness and her condition stabilizes. The Emergency Department provides her with Notice Of Privacy Practices (NOPP) and consent to treat.

   a) The hospital MUST tell Mrs. Goodman that her information will be put in the ***hospital directory*** and allow her an opportunity to object.

   b) The hospital MUST provide her with a ***Notice Of Privacy Practices***. Consent to treat is not a required HIPAA rule but is often a policy of the provider.

9. Mrs. Goodman is sent to the Radiology Department for an x-ray of her arm and chest and a CAT scan of her head to determine a possible cause of her fall.

   a) Radiology Department personnel must be ***authenticated*** by the system to access the patient database to add the report to Mrs. Goodman's medical record.

   b) The Privacy Rule does not limit sharing of medical information for ***reasons of treatment, payment, or health care operation***.

10. At break, an Emergency Department employee chats with other employees from various departments about their day. One of them mentions that the mayor's mother was brought in to the Emergency Department and had been treated very badly, maybe even abused. The staff wondered about her treatment and the mayor's upstanding position in the community. The discussion left those listening with questions about the mayor's family ethics. An OB nurse, having access to the patient database, used the computer system to look through Mrs. Goodman's information.

    a) The Privacy Rule requires immediate action to remedy any disclosure except for reasons of ***treatment, payment, or health care operations***. An employee should report concerns to her supervisor, not the individual, or law enforcement officials. The disclosure must be reported and corrected before it adversely affects the facility. Any whistle blowing should be encouraged and protected within the organization. Unchecked, the ramifications can reach all the way to the CEO of the organization.

b) All employees must comply with HIPAA Privacy Ruling with regard to disclosing PHI to anyone not treating the patient or face job termination.

11. Local authorities request an interview with the patient to see if allegations about the possible abuse are founded.

   a) Since HIPAA permits disclosure of protected health information to appropriate government authorities in cases of **victims of abuse, neglect, or domestic violence,** agents may question the patient.

12. Since the patient is the mayor's mother, word has gotten out and a local reporter comes to ask concerning her condition. He asks for her by name.

   a) HIPAA allows **release of directory information** to the public. This includes the patient's name, location in the facility, and description, in general terms, of the patient's condition. However, if Mrs. Goodman or the mayor has asked that her information NOT be included in the directory, the press or other public will not be given any information about the patient. This includes confirming whether or not she is in the hospital.

13. Mrs. Goodman's daughter finds out her mother is at the hospital and calls the hospital asking about her condition.

   a) **HIPAA ruling is not very clear about disclosure of information to family members**. Care must be given to ensure that the individual is really who they claim to be. If the hospital staff person personally knows the individual, then more information may be shared than if the person is not family. Each facility must define the policy that best fits their situation.

14. The next day, Mrs. Goodman's clergy comes to the hospital to visit parishioners. He stops at the information desk to request a list of members of his denomination that are listed as inpatients.

   a) Any patient who has registered under a religious denomination is placed on the list by denomination. If they have not chosen to "opt-out" of the **hospital directory,** their name, location, and general condition may be included on the list available to the clergy member.

15. Software in the Emergency Department searches for candidates for a statewide research study about treatment of elderly by family and neighbors. A research coordinator arrives in the Emergency Department, obtains an informed consent, and starts the research protocol.

    a) Mrs. Goodman's authorization for participation in the ***research study*** is required under FDA regulations, not HIPAA.

    b) Clinical ***research studies*** can access patient information without authorization provided that an Institutional Review Board (IRB) or Privacy Board has approved the research protocol.

    c) Researchers may obtain properly ***de-identified*** clinical data without authorization.

16. The hospital is a teaching hospital so medical interns participate in rounds with Dr. Eveready and report about Mrs. Goodman at "grand rounds."

    a) The ***definition of health care operations*** includes "conducting training programs in which students, trainees, or practitioners in areas of health-care learn under supervision to practice or improve their skills as health care providers."

    b) Medical students must be ***trained*** about HIPAA and the education must be documented.

    c) No special authorization is needed for this activity. It is permitted under ***"normal health care operations."***

17. Dr. Eveready consults with the resident psychologist, Dr. Wise, regarding the patient's status and possible modification of meds to stabilize her condition if lab tests deem that necessary.

    a) HIPAA does not limit disclosure of ***protected health information*** when it is for the treatment of a patient.

18. The Patient Accounts Department contacts Mrs. Goodman's health plan via online services to verify her eligibility using ANSI X12N 270 and receives a response using ANSI X12N 271 that her coverage is current and benefits provide for emergency care of her fracture.

    a) The eligibility inquiry and response must follow the ***designated ANSI X12 standard format.***

    b) The health plan, as a covered entity, may request ***minimum necessary*** information to process the request.

    c) Specific authorization is not required since use of ***protected health information*** is disclosed for payment of services.

    d) Any online transactions must be ***encrypted***.

19. Mrs. Goodman is admitted to the hospital for surgery to splint her arm by Dr. Bones, resident orthopedist, and then she will remain in the hospital for recovery. No other fracture is noted or any other serious injury.

    a) HIPAA allows ***business as usual*** as much as possible. There are no special authorization requirements for Dr. Bones to provide care.

b) Both doctors know each other through hospital contact. There is no requirement for Dr. Eveready to have a **Business Associate** agreement with Dr. Bones.

c) There is no limit to disclose only "**minimum necessary**" for purposes of treatment.

20. Dr. Bones dictates his operative report on Mrs. Goodman. After Dr. Bones signs using electronic signature software, the electronic report then becomes part of her medical record.

a) If a transcription service is used, a **Business Associate** contract must be in place.

b) Information sent across the Internet must be **encrypted**.

c) If transcription is done by hospital employees, those employees must be **trained** in HIPAA privacy and security and have the training documented.

d) Dr. Bones may use his electronic signature as long as the system **authenticates** him, integrity is maintained, and there is **nonrepudiation security**.

   i) Nonrepudiation: a 100% certainty that the physician did sign the document making it legal. Conversely, it cannot be proven that the physician did not sign the report/document. The document is undeniably authentic.

21. Dr. Eveready dictates Emergency Department notes and identifies the diagnoses and procedures performed. A copy is placed in Dr. Eveready's records also for teaching purposes.

a) A teaching file must contain **minimum necessary** information needed for teaching purposes.

22. The Health Information Management Department (Medical Records) receives patient information and abstracts information for medical record and billing purposes.

a) Disclosure of protected health information is permitted for **purposes of treatment, payment, and health care operations**.

23. The Patient Accounts Department submits a bill to the patient's insurance company electronically.

a) This transmission is a **designated ANSI X12 standard transaction**, N 837 Health Care Claim: Institutional, compliant with HIPAA transaction using **designated code sets** and **identifier standards**. The insurance company or health plan must accept the bill in this format, and cannot deny payment because it was received electronically.

b) The hospital may request status of the claim using a **standardized transmission request** ANSI X12N 276. The health plan must reply using the **standardized transmission reply** format, ANSI X12N 277.

   c) Payment will most likely be processed electronically using ***designated ANSI X12 standard format*** N 835 Health Care Claim Payment/Advice into the hospital's account if there is nothing noted on the claim that would need review.

24. The Hospital Foundation, following its usual custom, and considering the patient is the mother of the town mayor, requests a contribution from the prominent family for expansion of the Emergency Department facility.

   a) HIPAA rules permit this use of ***protected health information*** provided that notification of this type of use is included in its ***Notice of Privacy Practices***.

   b) The family may '***opt-out***' for future contact and this must be included in the ***Notice of Privacy Practices***.

25. Mr. Goodman, the mayor, is curious about what is written on his mother's medical record and requests a copy from the hospital to review. He has been named as "power of attorney for health care" for his mother.

   a) Patients or their representatives have the right to review and obtain a copy of a "***designated record set***" for as long as the ***Covered Entity*** maintains the information. The information disclosed must be defined as to the extent of disclosure request (designated) such as specific dates and types of information. A ***designated record set*** from a provider might contain medical records or billing records. Information from a health plan might include enrollment records, payment records, claims adjudication records, or case management records.

   b) There is <u>no automatic right to access</u> for psychotherapy notes; information in criminal, civil, or administrative action; or protected health information exempted by Clinical Laboratory Improvement Amendments (CLIA).

   c) A ***Covered Entity*** must act upon a request for information within 30 days or 60 days if the information is off-site.

26. The mayor requests that the Health Information Management Department disclose to him who has received outside access to his mother's medical record.

   a) The ***Covered Entity*** must act on a request within 60 days with a possible 30-day extension.

   b) ***Written accounting of disclosures of protected health information*** must include date of disclosure, person to whom the information was disclosed, brief description of information disclosed, and a copy of the authorization.

   c) ***Written accounting of disclosures of protected health information*** are provided free once per year; charges may be included if more requests are received.

    d) Documentation of ***disclosures of protected health information*** must be maintained for six years.

27. Mr. Goodman asks to have the record changed because he believes it is not correct.

    a) Individuals, or their representatives, have the right to ***request to amend***, not change, as long as the ***Covered Entity*** maintains the information.

    b) The ***Covered Entity*** may require a written request for rationale for the amendment and must act within 60 days of the request.

    c) If request is granted, the ***Covered Entity*** must:

        i) <u>Notify the individual</u> that the amendment was accepted

        ii) <u>Inform relevant person(s)</u> identified by the individual of the amendment

28. The hospital, after reviewing the request and a discussion with Dr. Eveready, denies the request to amend the medical record.

    a) The ***Covered Entity*** may deny a request if protected health information:

        i) Was not created by the ***Covered Entity***

        ii) Is not part of the ***designated record set*** requested

        iii) Was not available for inspection

        iv) Is accurate and complete

    b) The ***Covered Entity*** may prepare a rebuttal statement to the individual's statement of disagreement and must give a copy to the individual.

29. A local hospice organization has a doctoral student researching treatment of the elderly. The student requests information on all elderly patients brought to the Emergency Department for treatment of any kind over the past year.

    a) This information may be released without patient authorization if it is ***de-identified.***

        i) To be "***de-identified***" it cannot contain any of 18 specific identifiers of an individual and his relatives, employers, or household members.

        ii) If any identifiers remain, it may be released if a qualified statistician determines the risk of re-identification is very small.

        iii) Certain conditions in small communities may apply that require further ***de-identification*** to prevent deduced identification.

REFERENCES

Briggs, Bill. (2004, March). Taming the infrastructure beast. *Health Data Management*, 12(3), 37.

Ernst & Young. (2003, August 22). Advancing health in America. *Regulatory Advisory*, p. 2.

Piller, C. (2001, November 7). Web mishap: Kids' psychological files posted. *Los Angeles Times*, p. A 1.

DHS Surplus Sales Again Reveal Confidential Information. (2002, April). Associated Press.

Estate of Behringer v. Medical Center at Princeton, 249 NJ Super. 507, 1991.

Health Insurance Reform: Security Standards; Final Rule, 68 Fed. Reg. 8,333–8,381. (2003, February 20) (to codify 45 CFR Parts 160, 162, and 164).

Markoff, J. (1997, April 12). Privacy issue haunts sale of computer. *The New York Times,* p. 1:8.

Notice of Proposed Rule Making (NPRM): Security and Electronic Signature Standards. (last modified January 31, 2003). Centers for Medicare and Medicaid Services. Retrieved September 17, 2003 from http://www.cms.hhs.gov/hipaa/hipaa2/regulations/security/nprm/sec11.asp.

O'Harrow, R. (2000, December 9). Hacker accesses patient records. *The Washington Post,* p. E1.

Telehealth Update, Office for the Advancement of Telemedicine. (February 18, 2000). Retrieved September 17, 2003, from http://telehealth.hrsa.gov/pubs/privac/htm.

5

Unique Health Identifiers and Misconceptions

CHAPTER OUTLINE

Introduction

Reasons for Identification Numbers

    Employer Identifier

    Health Care Provider Identifier

    Health Plan Identifier

    Personal Identifier

What is Important to Know About HIPAA?

Misconceptions About HIPAA

Summary

KEY TERMS

check digit   National Provider Identifier (NPI)
Employer Identification Number (EIN)

THINK ABOUT IT

1. Identification numbers help keep covered entities clearly identified, but are not people's names just as good an identifier?

2. People have enough numbers to remember now. Do we need more? Would the inclusion of these new numbers eliminate others?

INTRODUCTION

The HIPAA law authorizes the Department of Health and Human Services (DHHS) to develop unique identifiers for all parties included in a health claim. The entities included are:

1. Health care providers
2. Health plans
3. Employers
4. Individual patients

This portion of HIPAA law has been prepared in parts. The first and easiest identifiers to standardize are the employer numbers. The next standardized identifier developed is the health care provider. After that comes the health plan unique identifier. Finally, there is the individual patient identifier, if the DHHS receives authority to develop it.

We will summarize the focus of the HIPAA law, since sometimes it is hard to remember the big picture. We can get lost in details. As the health care industry has wrestled with the rulings, some misconceptions about what HIPAA permits and does not permit have occurred. We will explore some of the most common myths that have arisen about HIPAA.

REASONS FOR IDENTIFICATION NUMBERS

Participants in the delivery of health care and health care payments include health care providers, health plans, employers, and the individuals receiving care. By standardizing health care transactions into codes rather than lengthy explanations or non-uniform names, the DHHS has greatly streamlined the transmissions and processing of transactions. This allows more information to be processed in a shorter time frame than if printed and mailed to the health plan. The codes bring a desirable efficiency. The last step in the Health Insurance Portability and Accountability Act of 1996 (HIPAA) was to uniformly identify the participants within the transaction according to a federal standard. This simplification eliminated the possible confusion of identity and removed distinctions between covered entities and employers. The law was written to require unique identifiers for all parties included in health care claims. At the time of this writing, the DHHS has developed the final rule for unique identifiers for employers and health care providers. Plans for unique identifiers for health plans will follow soon. Originally, the law included the development of unique health identifiers for individuals. The DHHS and Congress currently have postponed the development of the individual identifiers due to personal privacy concerns (Fact Sheet, 2003). There are some alternative options for unique identifiers that will possibly be considered.

Several organizations have been involved in determining the identifier standard to be adopted. These organizations are mentioned in the legislation. The important considerations are that the standard must improve the efficiency, effectiveness, and safety of the health care system. The standard must meet the needs of the health data standards user community. The code system must be consistent and uniform with other HIPAA standards in providing privacy and confidentiality.

Employer Identifier

The DHHS standardized employer identifiers first. When identifying an employer in a standard transaction as defined under HIPAA Transaction and Code Set Ruling, the Standard Unique Employer Identifier (SUEI) must be used. This identifier is not required for most claim forms generated by the health care provider. The DHHS defined this identifier to be the Employer Identification Number (EIN) issued by the Internal Revenue Service (IRS) under the authority of the Department of the Treasury. This standard was adopted after consultation with several organizations responsible for developing the transaction standards. They included the National Uniform Billing Committee (NUBC), the National Uniform Claim Committee (NUCC), the Workgroup for Electronic Data Interchange (WEDI), and the American Dental Association (ADA). The specific focus of these groups was explained in Chapter 3.

The DHHS issued the final rule regarding SUEI on July 30, 2002. The ruling issued July 2002 focused on employers. Employers were the first to be issued a uniform coding system. The employer of a patient or a patient's dependent was made responsible to ensure enrollment status in the employer's particular health plan. The standard adopted is the EIN. Those small employers who provide health care coverage and use a social security number (SSN) as their tax identification number (TIN) need to secure an EIN for use of the electronic transactions.

The **Employer Identification Number (EIN)** is a nine-digit code with a hyphen after the second digit: 00–0000000. This is the number that appears on the IRS Form W-2, Wage and Tax Statement, and on the employee's tax form. The IRS defined the format of two digits, a hyphen, and seven more digits. The first two digits of the employer identification number reflect the issuing Internal Revenue district. The rest of the numbers are unique identifiers with no "intelligence," that is, there is nothing to indicate a specific employer. Because most employers already have an employer identification number, the shift to adoption for HIPAA was relatively easy. A sole proprietor who has no employees or who files no excise or pension tax returns is the only businessperson who does not need to have an EIN as the taxpayer identifying number (Health Insurance Reform, 2002).

The use for this identifier is *required* when used between health plans and employers with regard to enrollment and disenrollment in a health plan. This is when ASC X12N 834—Benefit Enrollment and Maintenance in a Health Plan transaction is used. This transaction identifies the sponsor of the health plan when the sponsor is a self-insured employer. Other uses of the employer identification number (EIN) are *situational*—depending if the unique employer must be identified. Most uses do not involve the health care provider.

Presently, there are four *situational* uses of the standard unique employer identifier in the electronic transactions:

1. X12N 270/271 Transaction—Health Care Eligibility Benefit Inquiry and Response. Generally the health plan and employer communicate this information and the health care provider is not involved. The information is to verify that an employee is participating in the employer's group health plan. It is not protected health information (PHI), so HIPAA law does not apply.

2. X12N 276/277—Health Care Claim Status Request/Response. Employers identify themselves as the source of information about the eligibility of individuals in a worker's compensation claim. This is a situational use because the employer is not a covered entity and PHI is not transmitted. Most health care providers will have a relationship with the employer to treat worker's compensation cases and may already know the EIN.

3. X12N 834—Benefit Enrollment and Maintenance in a Health Plan. Use of the EIN is *situational* when used to identify the employer of a person covered under a health plan when that employer is *not* the sponsor. This differs from the *required* use explained above.

4. X12N 820—Health Plan Premium Payments. Employers use their EIN to identify themselves in transactions when enrolling or disenrolling their employees in a health plan. This transaction was not mentioned in Chapter 3 because this does not involve the health care provider.

Compliance to the above ruling for SUEI must be no later than July 30, 2004. Compliance for covered entities include all health care providers, health plans, and health care clearinghouses. Small health plans have another year—until August 1, 2005, to comply. Enforcement of this ruling has not been outlined as yet.

Health Care Provider Identifier

All health care providers have at least one identifier. Many providers have several. Medicare has issued a number. Medicaid organizations have issued another. Health plans have often issued their own identifier to be used on their claims. The National Provider Identifier as developed by the Centers for Medicare and Medicaid Service (CMS) will *replace all of these currently used identifiers*. The Unique Physician Identification Numbers (UPIN) contains "intelligence," meaning that information can be determined just by knowing the position format of the code. Those providers who have a Health Industry Number (HIN) will also need to apply for a National Provider Identifier (NPI). These HINs also contain "intelligence" about an entity. Licensed pharmacies are assigned a seven-digit identifier by the National Association of Boards of Pharmacy (NABP). This identifier has "intelligence" embedded in the code identifying the state where the pharmacy is located. Many health care providers currently use a National Provider Identifier (NPI). The HIPAA ruling has the same name *but is not the same identifier*. Every health care provider will need to apply for a NPI number through the National Provider System under the HIPAA regulations.

The DHHS has had input from many organizations to define the best identifier for providers of health care. The final rule has been issued January 23, 2004, and is effective May 23, 2004. The NUBC, which oversees hospital billing forms, UB-92, has had input into the adoption. Also the ADA, the NUCC (the group that reviews changes to the provider insurance claims on HCFA-1500), and the Workgroup for Electronic Data Interchange (WEDI) have sent recommendations to the secretary of the DHHS. They find that the NPI maintained by the CMS fits the requirements listed above.

The **National Provider Identifier (NPI)** is a 10-digit number system with the last digit being a **check digit**. A check digit provides a means to check that the number is accurate. An algorithm sums the nine digits and uses the ones number as the check. If numbers are transposed or entered in error, the check digit will not match and an error will be spotted. The International Standards Organization (ISO), which certifies many international and national businesses, uses the check digit in many standardized transactions. The NPI contains no embedded information about the provider that could identify the entity. The identifier will be able to accommodate all types of health care providers; for example, physicians, hospitals, licensed practitioners, suppliers of medical equipment, group practices, pharmacies, and certain non-institutional providers such as ambulance companies. The CMS believes that any identifier adopted must be capable of at least 100 million unique identifiers. This system is estimated to meet the needs of the United States for about 200 years.

The deadline for compliance has been set for three years after publication of the Final Rule. The Final Rule is effective May 23, 2004. The date for compliance is May 23, 2007, and small health plans have an additional year, to May 23, 2008, in order to comply.

Health Plan Identifier

Each health plan will also have a unique identifier to go along with the identifiers for each health care provider and employer that uses standardized transactions. The development of this standard is under the direction of the same committees that designated the standards for employers and providers of health care. The unique identifier for health plans is suggested to be the same as for employers—EIN, but the DHHS has not made any official decision as yet.

The details of the proposed rules for the Health Plan Identifier were not available as of this writing. The DHHS projects that this proposed rule will be issued sometime during the latter months of the 2004 calendar year.

Personal Identifier

Several organizations have begun to develop systems to identify individuals. The idea of a national identifier for each individual who may visit an institution for some type of health care is quite controversial. There are many ramifications to issuing every person in the United States a unique identification number. The very idea hints of invasion of personal privacy by governmental organizations to an even greater degree than currently exists. Imagine the many entities that might have health information about one patient: a primary care physician, several specialists, anesthesiologist, laboratory, hospital, pharmacist, durable medical equipment supplier, clinic, and mail order prescription provider just to treat one ailment. If records were to be interconnected, each of these providers would be linked to the one personal identifier.

Concerns about a personal identifier include:

1. Confidentiality and privacy concerns
2. Choice of the individual identifier—that it is truly unique
3. Legal protection of the information
4. The costs associated with moving to a new identifier
5. Who should pay for the costs of the transition
6. Issues dealing with accurate implementation of patient records by all entities. (Identifiers, 2004).

Even though legislation originally mandated this type of identifier, plans for implementation by the DHHS are moving very slowly at this time. The DHHS has published a white paper and has opened up the opportunity for discussion of this issue. Public comment has been encouraged. The DHHS is moving very, very slowly toward implementing unique health identifiers for individuals.

There are two very good reasons to have individual identifiers:

1. The quality of health care would be enhanced since there would be an accurate and rapid identification of an individual's health record spanning all providers.
2. With one coordinated location for all health information physicians would be able to coordinate medications prescribed by other providers and avoid allergic reactions to drugs and adverse drug interactions (Davidson and Holtz, 1998).

Several organizations are developing plans to establish a unique identifier for patients for possible future use (Unique Identifiers, 2004). There is information about seven possible systems that could be considered:

1. Standard Guide for Properties of a Universal Health Identifier (UHID)
2. Social Security Number (SSN)
3. Biometrics ID
4. Directory Service
5. Personal Immutable Properties
6. Patient Identification System based on existing Medical Record Number and Practitioner Prefix
7. Public-Key—Private-Key Cryptography Method

The current practice of identifying individuals consists of a medical record number or alphanumeric code issued by the individual provider organization. This is unique to the entity and not transferable to other systems. Some software vendors have explored developing a means to use these medical record numbers combined with a provider number to come up with a Corporate Master Patient Index. This system does not have much validity to be nationalized. The other identification systems listed above have more potential should the DHHS choose to adopt a standard. We will summarize each system.

Standard Guide for Properties of a Universal Health Identifier (UHID) is a standard being developed by the American Society for Testing and Materials (ASTM). The scheme of the identifier consists of a sequential identifier, a delimiter, check digits, and an encryption scheme to support data security. This system allows for automatically linking to various computer-based records. It supports data security of privileged clinical information and uses technology to keep operating costs to a minimum. It is reported that two veterans' hospitals are now implementing this system.

The Social Security Number (SSN) was originally planned to function only for the Social Security Administration. It has become a personal identifier with many applications including use by local, state, and federal authorities, financial institutions, and many consumer organizations. There are a number of issues that would eliminate this system from being unique:

❖ Social Security Numbers are not unique
❖ They lack check-digits
❖ There is significant level for error
❖ There are privacy and confidentiality risks
❖ They lack legal protection; they lack capacity for future growth
❖ They lack a mechanism for emergency use
❖ There is no provision for non-citizens

The Computer-based Record Institute (CPRI) is exploring using a modified SSN to include check digits and an encryption scheme.

Biometrics ID may use fingerprint, retinal pattern analysis, voice pattern identification, and DNA analysis as possible identifiers. There are law enforcement and immigration departments who use some of the biometric identification methods already. At present there are no standards, procedures, or guidelines for this type of use in the health care industry. Concerns for this identification system relate to organ transplant, amputation, and diseases affecting organs used for identification such as retinopathy affecting retinal pattern analysis.

A **Directory Service** is a proposal being developed by the Mitre Corporation. The Mitre Corporation is working to provide linkages with existing patient identifiers to allow connections across computer systems. They propose including social characteristics such as name, social security number, address, driver's license, and so on with human characteristics like finger prints, and retina scans. They propose using these with other groupings such as gender, race, and identification data at the current point of care. By connecting all of these identifiers electronically to other point of care locations information could be exchanged with a great accuracy. This is only being explored and is not in practice anywhere. Costs to implement this type of identification would be considerable.

Physicians at Mayo Clinic are considering **Personal Immutable Properties**. Their proposal consists of a series of three universal immutable values plus a check digit. The three values are a seven-digit date of birth field, a six-digit place of birth code, a five-digit sequence code (to separate individuals born on the same date in the same geographic area), and a single-check digit. This would be called a Unique Patient Identifier (UPI).

Patient Identification System based on existing Medical Record Number and Practitioner Prefix is a system proposed by the Medical Records Institute. This patient identification number uses the provider institution's patient medical record number with a provider number as prefix. This use of already defined numbers eliminates the cost of creating a new patient numbering system. The unique provider number would identify the location of the patient database and the medical record number would identify the patient's record with that database. This system allows the patient to designate a practitioner of choice to be the curator or the gateway to connect other data and update information.

The **Public-Key—Private-Key Cryptography Method** is a method being proposed by a doctor working with the Massachusetts Institute of Technology. This system of identifiers uses smart cards or keys and computers for accessing patient information. Two keys would be necessary to allow arbitrary messages to be encoded and decoded. The two keys would contain mathematical functions that are inverses to each other. One key is a patient private-key. The other is an organizational/provider-key. Together they generate and maintain identifiers that are specific and unique to the organization and individual patients within that organization. An umbrella organization would handle the patient private-keys via an ID server. The patient will have the public-key of the organization. With this concept, outside organizations requesting information would only gain access with the private-key of the patient. This plan depends heavily on computer technology.

These are possible solutions to the unique health identifiers as directed in the HIPAA law of 1996. The DHHS has stated that so far they are not moving in the direction to define *any standards* for individuals.

WHAT IS IMPORTANT TO KNOW ABOUT HIPAA?

The Congress directed the DHHS to write rulings mandating that all providers of health care, all health plans, and all health care clearinghouses adhere:

1. to a uniform set of standards to *ensure the privacy* of an individual's health care information,
2. to make it *easier for people* who move to another job to be able *to continue or begin health insurance coverage*,
3. to *standardize electronic transactions* by developing code sets and identifiers to be used,
4. to keep the electronic data containing *health information secure from adverse events or a break in security*.

Efficiency and uniformity have been the goal of the Title II rulings. That is the reason for calling it "Administrative Simplification." This causes changes to varying degrees for the covered entities involved. Facilities who handle data electronically within their organizations are realizing savings in turnaround time to receive payment for services, increased revenue from more efficient methods of conducting business, and greater patient confidence in the provider to keep their best interests in mind. The DHHS will need to modify their rulings to adjust to new challenges. The DHHS has promised this will happen. Any ruling will stand for 24 months. It may be modified or changed after that, as it seems necessary. Those responsible for compliance such as the HIPAA Officer need to routinely check with the DHHS's web site or other government sources to maintain compliance. Modifications are already being issued. Access to the department's website is a valuable part of the HIPAA Officer's job description. See Appendix A for listing of helpful website addresses.

Misconceptions About HIPAA

With new rulings come many ideas about what they really mean. Since the spring of 2003, many rumors have circulated about what HIPAA law really says and what it does not say. We will explain a few common misconceptions and how compliance with HIPAA really works. Also, note that the acronym is not "HIPPO" as in hippopotamus. This is the image many people have gotten when first considering the extent of the HIPAA ruling—that it is as large and bulky as a hippopotamus.

A. Myth—Appointment reminders: *To protect the privacy of PHI many receptionists were very concerned about leaving a voice mail reminder of a doctor's appointment. Any information that might be heard by someone other than the patient was a likely unauthorized disclosure. Some offices stopped phoning their patients completely. Some stopped sending postcard reminders. Others did not change procedures at all, hoping nothing would be said.*

Proper response: All information is to be kept to the "minimum necessary" as outlined in the Privacy Ruling. There is nothing wrong with leaving voice mail to remind patients of an upcoming appointment. Date, time, and the name of the doctor do not disclose health information. Even when the doctor is a particular specialist or a psychologist, this information will not disclose protected information to unauthorized individuals. Advise patients to call the office prior to the appointment if the patient has questions. This same guidance applies to postcard reminders.

B. Myth—Prescription pickup: *Family members were afraid that only the patient would be able to pick up prescriptions at the local pharmacy.*

Proper response: Clearly a pharmacist is not to give prescriptions to just anyone who walks up to their counter. Patients may not be able to travel to a pharmacy or complete the paperwork required to receive their medications. Under HIPAA regulation, a family member or other individual may act on the patient's behalf to pick up medications, medical supplies, X-ray films, or other forms of PHI. The DHHS issued guidance on this topic in a press release on July 6, 2001, stating that "the rule allows a friend or relative to pick up a patient's prescription at the pharmacy." The health care provider is to use professional judgment and common practice to determine if releasing the medication, supplies, or other items is in the patient's best interest. Verification of identity is a reasonable precaution.

C. Myth about discussing patient information with family members—*A hospital or physician cannot share any information with the patient's family without the patient's written consent.*

Proper response: The Privacy Rule permits a health care provider to "disclose to a family member, other relative, or a close personal friend of the individual" medical information directly pertaining to the person's involvement with the patient, the patient's care, or for payment related to the patient's care. A health care professional may receive verbal consent from the patient when discussing patient care with the family member. If a family member is present and the patient does not object, the physician can infer that the patient is giving consent for the private discussion of health care. In situations where the patient is unable to give consent, the covered entity may determine whether the disclosure is in the patient's best interests. In each situation above, the permission verbally received, inferred, or the inability to authorize must be documented in the patient's medical record. Documentation is vital. A mantra for all health care workers would be: "Document, document, document." You cannot go wrong by documenting too much.

D. Myth—Refusal to sign the Notice Of Privacy Practice: *A patient refuses to sign the acknowledgment of receipt of the Notice Of Privacy Practices. Should the health care provider refuse to provide services?*

Proper response: The Privacy Rule requires that providers make a "good faith effort" to receive acknowledgment of the notice. The law does not give the provider the right to refuse services. Such offer of notice and the refusal to sign would be noted in the patient's record, but in no way does that deny them access to service or treatment. The signature of acknowledgment is not consent for treatment, nor is it authorization to release medical records so it cannot be interpreted to mean more than the intended limited scope.

E. Myth—Hospital patient list is eliminated: *Many people believe they can no longer find out the status of a friend who has been hospitalized. Some believed that the hospital directory listing was a violation of the Privacy Rule.*

Proper response: The Privacy Rule permits hospitals to maintain a listing of patients unless the patient has chosen to opt out. This option is to be given when the patient registers for admission. Information that may be disclosed is limited to their location in the facility, such as room and bed number, and their condition stated in general terms. This assumes that the friend asks for the patient by his full name and not just "someone named Bobby." The inquirer must know the full name.

F. Myth—Sharing of patient information between doctors: *Since consent and authorization were detailed in the NOPP, many providers assumed that nothing could be shared with a consulting physician without authorization.*

Proper response: The Privacy Rule permits freedom to share PHI among health care providers who are involved in the direct treatment of a patient without further authorization. Without this ability to discuss services or treatment of patients, the delivery of health care would be greatly impaired.

G. Myth—Medical records are separate from other information on file: *Patients can only receive information that pertains directly to their health care. This can also include financial reports regarding payment or non-payment of account. Financial information is the physician's and does not come under the Privacy Rule for patient copy.*

Proper response: Patients can request a copy of their medical record. The patient may also request a *designated record set* of billing information. Records such as copies of correspondence to a collection agency that the covered entity has on file are legitimate requests. The DHHS's Office of Civil Rights will help explain the patient's right to disclosure.

H. Myth—Members of clergy denied hospital information: *With the patient given the option to not reveal any information in the hospital directory, many felt that clergy members would not be able to have a list of patients who may be members of their parish.*

Proper response: Any patient who permits the facility to place their name in the directory may also be included on the list of patients who have listed their faith as the same denomination as the requesting clergy. The patient has the choice to opt out of this disclosure separately. Any policy more restrictive than this is an internal hospital policy rather than permitted HIPAA law.

I. Myth—Protected health information is disclosed in many new ways: *Patients received the NOPP. The list outlined when the HIPAA law allowed PHI to be disclosed and used. Many people felt this greatly increased the legal uses and disclosures of their PHI.*

Proper response: The DHHS mandates only two situations for disclosure: to the individual patient upon request and to the secretary of the DHHS for use in oversight investigations. Permitted disclosures have always been allowed for purposes such as incidents of possible abuse, neglect, domestic violence, national security, public health monitoring, and law enforcement. HIPAA does not conflict with or limit these permitted uses of disclosure.

J. Myth—Patients will sue health care providers for non-compliance: *The fear of many providers is now that patients have written notice of when, where, and why PHI may be used, patients will feel any infraction is permission to begin a law suit.*

Proper response: The HIPAA Privacy Rule does not give people the right to sue a provider. Instead, if a person feels that the privacy of their information has been violated and has not received a satisfactory reply, a complaint may be filed with the secretary of the DHHS through the Office of Civil Rights. The DHHS has the discretion to investigate the complaint. If the

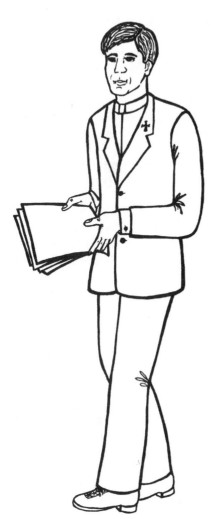

Figure 5-1 If a patient chooses to opt-out of the patient directory, clergy members may not receive a complete listing of their parishioners in the hospital.

health care provider is found to be non-compliant, the DHHS may impose civil penalties and if flagrant violations are found, file criminal charges. However, the DHHS seeks to promote education and voluntary compliance, and desires to work toward compliance rather than imposing penalties. It is very important for the provider to understand that violations are opportunities for education more than punishment.

K. Myth—The press is prohibited from receiving any public information from hospital personnel: *Members of the press will no longer be permitted any information about accident or crime victims from a hospital spokesperson.*

Proper response: Members of the press are to be treated just as any other person requesting information concerning a patient in the facility. Any patient may opt out of disclosing their name on the facility directory. When a patient does not want their name in a directory, they certainly do not want the provider's personnel talking to the press about their status. If the patient permits their name to be placed in the facility directory, the location and general condition can be released to the members of the press. If a state law restricts the hospital further, the state law takes precedence. Individual provider policy may be even more restrictive. Once a reporter receives patient information, the HIPAA law does not restrict the press in how they choose to convey the information given.

L. Myth—Faxing of health information is now prohibited: *Fax machines have been widely used to send health information between providers. With the HIPAA Privacy Rule, the possible disclosure of protected health information to unauthorized persons is punishable by law. Many facilities refuse to send any information by means of the fax machine.*

Proper response: Fax machines have truly made it a lot easier to send and receive information quickly. With that ease comes some very large risks of improper disclosure. The machine must be in a secure location away from unauthorized access. An audit trail or record must be kept to document that information was sent to the proper location. This record is to be kept for six years. A cover sheet is necessary with disclaimers that this fax is intended for the designated person only. The best protection is to call the receiving party, send the fax information, and then follow up with another phone call to confirm receipt of the information. Do not forget to log the confirmation.

Proper response when information is misdirected: If faxed health information is sent to the wrong fax number, immediate response is the best choice. Call the party that received the information and retrieve it if possible. If not retrievable, advise them to shred the papers immediately. Then make a notation in the patient's record of the error and what was done to remedy it. Notification of the patient should not be necessary unless sensitive medical information was disclosed without knowledge of who received the information.

M. Myth—Patient access to records you did not create: *Your office received reports from a referring doctor to assist with the treatment of a patient. That patient asks for a copy of his medical record. Do you include anything received from another doctor? Must the patient request the copy from the originating doctor?*

Proper response: Once your office receives protected medical information and includes it with your files, it becomes part of the medical record set of documents. These are to be included when a copy is requested. To claim that information from another source does not exist or that it is not part of the patient file denies that treatment and services were influenced by the information contained in the file.

SUMMARY

The DHHS has been instructed to provide national identifiers for each of the individuals and organizations that are named on a typical health insurance claim form. This list includes employers, physicians, health plans, and patients. Adoption of the patient identifier is not planned at this time due to privacy issues. The other identifiers are being published currently. The employer identifier came first—EIN issued by the Internal Revenue Service; next the physician identifier was proposed as the NPI. The identifier for health plans is currently in the development stage. The proposed ruling should be issued sometime in 2004.

The Title II HIPAA ruling called Administrative Simplification is the first nationwide legislation to reform the health care industry. Standardization makes it a lot easier for individually covered entities to communicate with each other since it does away with unique qualifications previously demanded by particular health plans. With new rulings come misconceptions about just how these rules are implemented. In all cases, the goal of HIPAA is to make reasonable changes so health care is improved and reimbursed in a more efficient manner.

END OF CHAPTER QUESTIONS

1. What four categories of identifiers has the HIPAA law mandated?

2. What is the designated identifier for employers to use in standard transactions?

3. What is the designated identifier for health care providers to use in standard transactions?

4. What identifier is the next to be issued by the DHHS (after January 2004)?

5. List three objections to patient identifiers.

6. List two ways that unique health identifiers for patients would benefit patients.

Scenarios

How would you answer?

The following scenarios have caused a lot of confusion as to the proper response. What is the proper HIPAA response?

1. A patient is recovering after a minor surgical procedure. After recovery, the patient waits to receive final discharge instructions. If the patient's relative or friend is present too, instead of requesting to speak alone with the patient, you say, "I'd like to talk about discharge instructions with your relative present because it is often best to have another pair of ears to hear this information." Have you covered the need for authorized disclosure of PHI?

2. A Patient Account worker calling to ask a patient about bill payments leaves a voice mail message on the patient's phone stating the doctor's office and phone number and explains that payment is due in full within three business days. Is this acceptable information to leave on voice mail?

3. A patient is referred to a collection agency for failure to pay a bill or a co-payment. The patient requests a copy of the letter from the physician's office but the office refuses. Is this refusal in compliance with the Privacy Ruling because a letter to a collection agency is not part of the medical care or treatment of the patient?

REFERENCES

Davidson, K. E., & Holtz, D. L. (1998, October). Do unique identifiers violate patient privacy? *Physician's News Digest, 11–12,* p. 8.

Fact Sheet—Administrative Simplification Under HIPAA: National Standards for Transactions, Security and Privacy. (2003, March 3). Department of Health and Human Services. Retrieved September 12, 2003 from http: www.hhs.gov/news/press/2002pres/hipaa.html.

Health Insurance Reform: Standard Unique Employer Identifier, 67 Fed. Reg. 38,009-38,020. (May 30, 2002) (to codify 45 CFR parts 160 and 162).

HIPAA Administrative Simplification: Standard Unique Health Identifier for Health Care Providers, 69 Fed. Reg. 3,434-3,469. (2004, January 23) (to codify 45 CFR Part 162).

Identifiers, Background papers. Retrieved February 23, 2004 from http://www.wedi.org/snip/public/articlesdetails~htm.

Unique Identifiers (including allowed uses). Retrieved February 25, 2004 html version of http://www.virtual.epm.br/material/healthcare/spanish/F_Refer3dd.pdf.

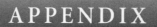

Resources for Further Information

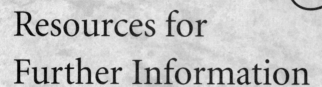

CENTERS FOR MEDICARE & MEDICAID SERVICES REGIONS

Region	CMS Regional Geographical Areas	Phone number
Atlanta	Alabama, Florida, Georgia, Kentucky, Mississippi, Tennessee, North Carolina, South Carolina	404-562-7427
Boston	Connecticut, Maine, Massachusetts, Vermont, New Hampshire, Rhode Island	617-565-1289
Chicago	Illinois, Indiana, Michigan, Minnesota, Ohio, Wisconsin	312-353-8583
Dallas	Arkansas, Louisiana, New Mexico, Oklahoma, Texas	214-767-6484
Denver	Colorado, Montana, North Dakota, South Dakota, Utah, Wyoming	303-844-7030
Kansas City	Iowa, Kansas, Missouri, Nebraska	816-426-5472
New York	New Jersey, New York, Puerto Rico, Virgin Islands	212-264-3885
Philadelphia	Delaware, District of Columbia, Maryland, Pennsylvania, Virginia, West Virginia	215-861-4259
San Francisco	American Samoa, Arizona, California, Guam, Nevada, Northern Mariana Islands, Hawaii	415-744-3674
Seattle	Alaska, Idaho, Oregon, Washington	206-615-2391

RELEVANT WEB SITES

Privacy Rule Resources—Chapter 2

1. Subscribe to HIPAA REGS listserv for notification via e-mail at www.cms.hhs.gov/ hipaa
2. Centers for Medicare and Medicaid Services for HIPAA information. www.cms.gov/ hipaa
3. Government Printing Office for Federal Register documents and original source documents. www.access.gpo.gov
4. The Office of Civil Rights (OCR). Responsible for overseeing compliance with the HIPAA privacy rulings. www.hhs.gov/ocr
5. Email questions to the Centers for Medicare and Medicaid Services. askhipaa@cms. hhs.gov
6. Centers for Medicare and Medicaid Services HIPAA HOTLINE: 1-866-282-0659
7. Department of Health and Human Services—This government website contains links to other government websites related to HIPAA Privacy, Transactions and Security. http://www.os.dhhs.gov
8. Health Privacy Project—The Health Privacy Project is dedicated to raising public awareness of the importance of ensuring health privacy so access and quality of health care are improved. http://www.healthprivacy.org
9. HIPAA Advisory Site—Provided by Phoenix Health Systems, an information technology consulting and outsourcing company. There are many areas providing current HIPAA information and an email subscription service. http://www.hipaadvisory.com

Transactions and Code Sets Resources—Chapter 3

10. Address for Food and Drug Administration: Food and Drug Administration Freedom of Information Office, HFI-35, 5600 Fishers Lane, Rockville, MD 20857, www.fda.gov
11. Government website for Designated Standard Maintenance Organizations: (DSMO) http://www.hipaa-dsmo.org

Names and websites for Designated Standard Maintenance Organizations (DSMO)

12. Accredited Standards Committee X12—Develops transmission standards for business and industry transactions. http://www.x12.org
13. Dental Content Committee of the American Dental Association—Develops dental procedures and Current Dental Terminology Version 4 codes. http://www.ada.org
14. Health Level Seven—Develops transaction standards for claims attachments. http:// www.hl7.org
15. National Council for Prescription Drug Programs—Designated to maintain listing of drugs and biologics for retail pharmacy drug transactions. http://www.ncpdp.org
16. National Uniform Billing Committee—Maintains standards for hospital billing form UB-92 http://www.nubc.org
17. National Uniform Claim Committee—Maintains standards for HCFA-1500 physician services insurance claims. http://www.nucc.org

Security Rule Resources—Chapter 4

18. Association for Electronic Health Care Transactions—AFECHT http://www. afehct.org
19. American Hospitals Association—AMA http://www.hospitalconnect.com
20. American Health Information Management Association—AHIMA http://www. ahima.org
21. American Health Lawyers Association—AHLA http://www.ahla.org
22. American Medical Informatics Association—AMIA http://www.amia.org
23. Department of Health and Human Services—DHHS http://aspe.os.dhhs.gov
24. Department of Health and Human Services—Data Council http://www.aspe.os.dhhs. gov/datacncl
25. Strategic National Implementation Process—WEDI/SNIP Workgroup for Electronic Data Interchange (WEDI) started the HIPAA project called Strategic National Implementation Process (SNIP). This group assists the implementation of standards for administrative simplification mandated by HIPAA. http://www.wedi.org/snip
26. Washington Publishing Company—WPC. The government source for implementation guides to all transactions. http://www.wpc-edi.com
27. National Infrastructure Protection Center (NIPC). Website dealing with security issues for information systems. http://www.nipc.gov

Identifiers Rule Resources—Chapter 5

28. HIPAA Administrative Simplification–Identifiers http://www.cms.hhs.gov/hipaa

B

Required and Addressable Security Standards

From Appendix A to Subpart C of Part 164, Security Standards, Matrix from Federal Register/Vol. 68, No.34 February 20,2003/Rules and Regulations, p. 8380.

SECTION: ADMINISTRATIVE SAFEGUARDS

Standard	Implementation Specification	Required/Addressable
Security Management Process	Risk Analysis	R
	Risk Management	R
	Sanction Policy	R
	Information System Activity Review	R
Assigned Security Responsibility		R
Workforce Security	Authorization and/or Supervision	A
	Workforce Clearance Procedure	A
	Termination Procedures	A
Information Access Management	Isolating Health Care Clearinghouse Functions	R
	Access Authorization	A
	Access Establishment and Modification	A
Security Awareness & Training	Security Reminders	A
	Protection from Malicious Software	A
	Log-in Monitoring	A
	Password Management	A

(continued)

Standard	Implementation Specification	Required/Addressable
Security Incident Procedures	Response and Reporting	R
Contingency Plan	Data Backup Plan	R
	Disaster Recovery Plan	R
	Emergency Mode Operation Plan	R
	Testing and Revision Procedures	A
	Applications and Data Criticality Analysis	A
Evaluation		R
Business Associate Contracts & Other Arrangements	Written Contract or Other Arrangement	R

SECTION: PHYSICAL SAFEGUARDS

Standard	Implementation Specification	Required/Addressable
Facility Access Controls	Contingency Operations	A
	Facility Security Plan	A
	Access Control and Validation Procedures	A
	Maintenance Records	A
Workstation Use		R
Workstation Security		R
Device and Media Controls	Disposal	R
	Media Re-Use	R
	Accountability	A
	Data Backup and Storage	A

SECTION: TECHNICAL SAFEGUARDS

Standard	Implementation Specification	Required/Addressable
Access Control	Unique User Identification	R
	Emergency Access Procedure	R
	Automatic Logoff	A
	Encryption and Decryption	A
Audit Controls		R
Integrity	Mechanism to Authenticate Electronic PHI	A
Person or Entity Authentication		R
Transmission Security	Integrity Controls	A
	Encryption	A

SECTION: ORGANIZATIONAL REQUIREMENTS

Business Associate Contracts or other arrangements: Required

SECTION: POLICIES AND PROCEDURES AND DOCUMENTATION REQUIREMENTS

Policies and Procedures: Required

    Time limit: required, retain for six years

    Availability: required, available to those responsible for implementing

    Updates: required, review periodically

C

Further Scenarios and Questions for Consideration

1. Can patients schedule appointments over the phone with my office, or is written authorization needed first?

2. My doctor performs surgery. Often we contact the hospital and other health care providers to collect pre-op information over the phone for the new patient so that we can determine if there are medical concerns to be addressed prior to surgery. The patient has not received our Privacy Notice as yet. Does the Privacy Rule prohibit this practice since the patient may not have given specific authorization to this health information?

3. When more than one doctor is treating a patient, is a signed authorization needed in order to send medical records to another provider?

4. Can a complete medical record be disclosed to another provider? What limits are necessary, if any?

5. At the hospital information desk, someone asks if her cousin is in the hospital. They give the last name of Johnson. Can the receptionist advise the visitors of the room number and condition of the patient?

6. Can a clergy find out more information about patients in the hospital than a friend of the patient?

7. A "relative" calls the office and asks for a copy of "Mom's" lab report to be faxed to her house to take to another doctor for a second opinion. Is this permitted under the Privacy Rule?

8. The District Attorney calls the office with a request that all documentation relating to a patient be released to her office. Is authorization needed? In what form?

9. An "auditor" from the Office of Inspector General comes to the office and requests billing records. What questions would the office worker ask to verify the validity of her claim?

10. A physician sends an individual's health plan coverage information to a laboratory that needs the information to bill for services it provided to the physician with respect to the individual. Is authorization needed?

11. A health care provider discloses PHI to a health plan for the plan's Health Plan Employer Data and Information Set (HEDIS) purposes. This health plan has a relationship with the individual who is the subject of the information. Is authorization needed?

12. A drug manufacturer received a list of patients from a health care provider. They reimbursed the provider for providing the list and then used that list to send discount coupons for a new anti-depressant medication directly to the patients. Is this considered marketing?

13. A pharmacy mails prescription refill reminders to patients, or contracts with a mail house to do so. Is this considered marketing?

14. An insurance agent sells a health insurance policy in person to a customer and proceeds to also market a casualty and life insurance policy as well. Is this considered marketing under the Privacy Rule?

15. An endocrinologist shares a patient's medical records with several behavior management programs to determine which program best suits the ongoing needs of the individual patient. Is this considered marketing?

16. A health plan sells a list of its members to a manufacturing company that sells blood glucose monitors. This manufacturer intends to send the plan's members brochures on the benefits of purchasing and using the monitors. Is this considered marketing?

17. Consider a mailing from a health insurer promoting a home and casualty insurance product offered by the same company. Is this considered marketing?

Glossary

The bracketed numbers refer to the chapter in which the term appears.

A

access [4]—the ability or the means necessary to read, write, modify, or communicate data/information or otherwise use any system resource.

adjudication [3]—the act of making a judicial decision or sentence.

administrative safeguards [4]—administrative actions, and policies and procedures, to manage the selection, development, implementation, and maintenance of security measures to protect electronic protected health information and to manage the conduct of the covered entity's workforce in relation to the protection of that information.

algorithm [4]—a step-by-step procedure for solving a problem or accomplishing a specific purpose.

ASC X12 Standards [3]—Accredited Standards Committee-developed uniform standards (X12) for inter-industry electronic exchange of business transactions-electronic data interchange (EDI).

audit trail(s) [4]—data collected and potentially used to facilitate a security audit, to include the "who" (login ID), what (read-only, modify, delete, add, etc.), and when (date/timestamp).

authentication [4]—the corroboration or confirmation that a person is the one claimed.

authorization [2]—written permission by the patient or the patient's personal representa-tive allowing the use or disclosure of specific protected health information for purposes other than treatment, payment, and health care operations or uses and disclosures permitted or required by the Privacy Rule.

B

biologic [3]—products used to make medicines

Business Associate(s) (BA) [2]—a person or organization that performs or assists a function or activity on behalf of a covered entity, but is not part of the covered entity's workforce. Functions may involve the use or disclosure of individually identifiable health information, including claims processing, data analysis, processing, administration, utilization review, quality assurance, billing, benefit management, practice management, re-pricing, or someone who provides legal, actuarial, accounting, consulting, accredita-tion, or financial services to or for a covered entity. A Business Associate can also be a covered entity in its own right.

C

check digit [5]—a check digit provides a means to check that the number is accurate. The usual algorithm is to add each of the digits in the number and use the ones digit in the check digit place.

code sets [3]—any set of codes used to encode data elements, such as tables of terms, medical concepts, medical diagnostic codes, or medical procedure codes. A code set includes the codes and the descriptors (words of description) of the codes.

consent [2]—permission granted by the patient or the patient's representative to use or disclose protected health information for purposes of treatment, payment, or health care operations.

contingency plan [4]—policies and procedures for responding to an emergency or other occurrence that damages systems containing electronic protected health information.

covered entity [2]—under HIPAA, this is a health plan, a health care clearinghouse, or a health care provider who transmits any health information in electronic form in connection with a HIPAA transaction.

crossover claim [3]—a Medicare claim that Medicare transmits electronically to the secondary coverage health plan, usually but not limited to Medicaid or Medigap plans.

D

de-identified health information [2]—health information that does not identify or provide a reasonable basis to identify an individual.

designated record set [2]—a group of related data maintained by or for a covered entity that includes the medical records and billing records about individuals maintained by or for a covered health care provider; the enrollment, payment, claims adjudication, and case or medical management record systems maintained by or for a health plan; used, in whole or in part, by or for the covered entity to make decisions about individuals. Disclosure of medical information must define or designate the extent of the disclosure, for example, the EKG tracing, or the complete medical records for encounter covering specified dates, or the employment status of a subscriber to a health plan.

disclosure [2] of protected health information (PHI)—the release, transfer, divulging of, or providing access to protected health information to an outside entity.

E

Electronic Data Interchange (EDI) [3]—computer-to-computer transmission of business information in a standard format

using national standard communications protocols.

emancipated minor [2]—a person younger than 18 years of age who lives independently, is totally self-supporting, is married or divorced, is a parent even if not married, or is in the military and possesses decision-making rights.

Employer Identification Number (EIN) [5]—the Employer Identification Number assigned by the Internal Revenue Service. The EIN is the taxpayer identifying number of an individual or other entity assigned as the taxpayer in tax returns and statements or other required documents explained in the Internal Revenue Code.

encryption [4]—the use of an algorithmic process to transform data into a format in which there is a low probability of assigning meaning without use of a confidential process or key; transforming confidential plain text into cipher text to protect it. Once encrypted, data can be stored or transmitted over unsecured lines.

etiology [3]—all causes of a disease or abnormal condition.

F

format [3]—those data elements that provide or control the enveloping or hierarchical structure, or assist in identifying data content of a transaction.

G

group health plan [1]—an employee welfare benefit plan that provides health coverage in the form of medical care and services through insurance, reimbursement, or other means for a group of employees and dependents. It may be sponsored by an employer or a union and includes private employer plans, federal governmental plans, non-federal governmental plans, and church plans.

H

Health Care (Financing Administration) Procedure Coding System (HCPCS) [3]—a coding system maintained by the Centers for Medicare and Medicaid Services (CMS) for non-physician services such as, but not limited to, medical supplies, orthotic and prosthetic devices, and durable medical equipment.

health care clearinghouse [1]—a public or private entity that does either of the following (entities, including but not limited to, billing services, re-pricing companies, community health management information systems or community health information systems, and "value-added" networks and switches are health care clearinghouses if they perform these functions): (1) processes or facilitates the processing of information received from another entity in a nonstandard format or containing nonstandard data content into standard data elements or a standard transaction; (2) receives a standard transaction from another entity and processes or facilitates the processing of information into nonstandard format or nonstandard data content for a receiving entity.

health care operations [2]—certain administrative, financial, legal, and quality improvement activities of a covered entity that are necessary to run its business and to support the core functions of treatment and payment.

health care provider [1]—a provider of medical or other health services and any other person who furnishes, bills, or is paid for health care in the normal course of business.

Health Insurance Portability and Accountability Act of 1996 (HIPAA) [1]—a federal law that allows persons to qualify immediately for comparable health insurance coverage when they change their employment relationships. Title II, subtitle F, of HIPAA gives the DHHS the authority to mandate the use of standards for the electronic exchange of health care data; to specify what medical and administrative code sets should be used within those standards; to require the use of national identification systems for health care patients, providers, payers (or plans), and employers (or sponsors); and to specify the types of measures required to protect the security and privacy of personally identifiable health care information. Also known as the Kennedy-Kassebaum Bill, the Kassebaum-Kennedy Bill, K2, or Public Law 104-191.

health plan [2]—an entity that assumes the risk of paying for part or all medical treatments,

that is, uninsured patient, self-insured employer, payer, or HMO as outlined in their policy coverage. Examples of various plans are: group health plans, health insurance issuer, health maintenance organization, Part A or Part B of Medicare, Medicaid program, Medicare supplemental policy, long-term care policy, employee welfare benefit plan, health care program for active military personnel, veterans health care program (CHAMPVA), Civilian Health and Medical Program of the Uniformed Services (CHAMPUS), Indian health service program, Federal Employees Health Benefit Plan.

HIPAA Officer [2]—person responsible at each covered entity to keep abreast of HIPAA rulings and in turn train and educate rest of the workforce in how to comply with the rulings.

I

incidental disclosure [2]—a disclosure of individually identifiable health information (IIHI) as a result of or as "incident to" otherwise permitted use or disclosure.

individually identifiable health information (IIHI) [2]—any protected health information about an individual that can possibly identify that individual with the medical information included.

information system [4]—an interconnected set of information resources under the same direct management control that shares common functionality. A system normally includes hardware, software, information, data, applications, communications, and people.

infrastructure [4]—the underlying foundation or basic framework (as of a system or organization) including hardwired and wireless networks, servers, routers, and other hardware and software that direct information system commands and responses, and transport and store data.

integrity [4]—the property that data or information have not been altered or destroyed in an unauthorized manner.

L

limited data set [2]—protected health information that excludes the following direct identifiers of the individual or of relatives, employers, or household members of the individual. Examples are names, postal address information, telephone numbers, fax numbers, electronic mail addresses, social security numbers, medical record numbers, health plan beneficiary numbers, account numbers, certificate and license numbers, vehicle identifiers and serial numbers, license plate numbers, device identifiers and serial numbers, biometric identifiers, and full face photographic images or comparable images.

M

marketing [2]—any communication about a product or service that encourages recipients to purchase or use the product or service unless the communication is used (1) to describe a health-related product or service provided by or included in the plan of benefits of the covered entity; (2) for treatment of the individual; (3) for case management or care coordination for the individual or to recommend alternative treatments, therapies, health care providers, or setting of care to the individual.

Medical Savings Account (MSA) [1]—a tax-sheltered savings account similar to an IRA, but earmarked for medical expenses only. Deposits are 100% tax-deductible for the self-employed and can be easily withdrawn by check or debit card to pay routine medical bills with tax-free dollars.

minimum necessary [2]—when using or disclosing protected health information or when requesting protected health information from a covered entity, reasonable efforts must be made to limit protected health information to only that which is necessary to accomplish the intended purposes of the use, disclosure, or request.

N

National Provider Identifier (NPI) [5]—a system for uniquely identifying all providers of health care services, supplies, and equipment. A term proposed by the secretary of the DHHS as the standard identifier for health care providers.

need-to-know [2]—a security principle stating that a user should have access only to the data he or she needs to perform a particular function.

nomenclature [3]—a designation; the act or process of naming.

nonrepudiation security [4]—a method by which the sender of data is provided with proof of delivery and the recipient is assured of the sender's identity, so that neither can later deny having processed the data.

O

orthotic [3]—a support or brace for weak or ineffective joints or muscles.

P

password [4]—confidential numeric and/or character string used in conjunction with a User ID to verify the identity of the individual attempting to gain access to a computer system.

physical safeguards [4]—physical measures, policies, and procedures to protect a covered entity's electronic information systems and related buildings and equipment from natural and environmental hazards and unauthorized intrusion.

privacy [1]—an individual's claim to control the use and disclosure of personal information. This claim is backed by the societal value representing that claim.

Protected Health Information (PHI) [2]—individually identifiable health information transmitted or maintained in any form or medium, which is held by a covered entity or its business associate that: (1) identifies the individual or offers a reasonable basis for identification; (2) is created or received by a covered entity or an employer; (3) relates to a past, present, or future physical or mental condition, provision of health care, or payment for health care.

protocol [3]—a set of conventions governing the treatment and especially the formatting of data in an electronic communications system; a code prescribing strict adherence to correct etiquette and precedence.

Provider Taxonomy Code [3]—a standard administrative code set for identifying the provider type and area of specialization for all health care providers. This will be discontinued with a new system of identifying providers under HIPAA.

psychotherapy notes [2]—notes recorded (in any medium) by a health care provider who is a mental health professional documenting or analyzing the contents of conversation during a private counseling session or a group, joint, or family counseling session and that are separate from the rest of the individual's medical record. Psychotherapy notes exclude prescriptions, monitoring, counseling sessions start and stop times, the modalities and frequencies of treatment furnished, results of clinical tests, and any summary of the following items: diagnosis, functional status, the treatment plan, symptoms, prognosis, and progress to date.

R

risk [4]—the impact and likelihood of an adverse event; the possibility of harm or loss to any software, information, hardware, administrative, physical, communications, or personnel resource within an automated information system or activity.

risk analysis [4]—a process whereby cost-effective security/control measures may be selected by balancing the cost of various security/control measures against the losses that would be expected if these measures were not in place.

risk management [4]—the ongoing process that assesses the risk to electronic information resources and the information itself in order to determine adequate security measures to offset the threats to and vulnerabilities of protected health information.

S

security [4] of protected health information (PHI)—the safeguards (administrative, technical, or physical) in an information system that protect it and its information against unauthorized disclosure, and limit access to authorized users in accordance with an established policy.

security incident [4]—the attempted or successful unauthorized access, use, disclosure, modification, or destruction of information or interference with system operations in an information system.

subscriber [3]—the person whose name is listed in the health insurance policy.

T

technical safeguards [4]—the technology and the policy and procedures for its use that protect electronic protected health information and control access to it.

Trading Partner [3]—external entity, with whom business is conducted, that is, customer. This relationship can be formalized via a Trading Partner Agreement. (Note: a Trading Partner or an entity for some purposes, may be a business associate of that same entity for other purposes.)

Trading Part Agreement (TPA) [3]—an agreement related to the exchange of information in electronic transactions, whether the agreement is distinct or part of a larger agreement, between each party to the agreement. (For example, a Trading Partner Agreement may specify, among other things, the duties and responsibilities of each party to the agreement in conducting a standard transaction.)

transaction [1]—under HIPAA this is the exchange of information between two parties to carry out financial or administrative activities related to health care.

treatment [2]—the provision, coordination, or management of health care and related services for an individual by one or more health care providers or by a health care provider with a third party, including consultation between health care providers regarding a patient and referral of a patient from one health care provider to another.

U

use [2] of protected health information (PHI)—the sharing, employment, application, utilization, examination, or analysis of individually identifiable health information (IIHI) within an entity that maintains such information.

user [4]—a person or entity with authorized access.

W

workforce [2]—employees, volunteers, trainees, and other persons under the direct control of a covered entity, whether or not they are paid by the covered entity.

workstation [4]—an electronic computing device, for example, a laptop or desktop computer, or any other device that performs similar functions, and electronic media stored in its immediate environment.

X

X12N [3]—a subcommittee of ASC/X12 that defines Electronic Data Interchange (EDI) standards for the insurance industry.

Index

access, 59, 73, 98
Accredited Standards Committee (ASC), 36, 38, 42
algorithms, 70
American Dental Association (ADA), 89, 91
American Health Information Management Association (AHIMA), 39, 40
American Medical Association (AMA), 41, 42
American National Standards Institute (ANSI), 42
American Society for Testing and Materials (ASTM), 92
appointment reminders, 95
Archer, Bill, 4
ASC X12 standards, 38, 42–43, 53, 89–90
architecture, 43, 45–46
ASC X12N 820, Health Plan Premium Payments, 90
ASC X12N 837, Health Care Claim, 43, 45, 51
ASC X12N 270, Health Care Eligibility Benefit Inquiry, 43, 45, 90
ASC X12N 271, Health Care Eligibility Benefit Response, 43, 45, 90
ASC X12N 276, Health Care Claim Status Request, 43, 45, 90
ASC X12N 277, Health Care Claim Status Response, 43, 45, 90
ASC X12N 278, Health Care Services Review, 43, 45
ASC X12N 834, Benefit Enrollment and Maintenance, 43, 45–46, 89, 90

ASC X12N 835, Health Care Claim Payment/Advice, 43, 46, 51
claim form versions, 45–46
data overview, 43
limitation to claims encounters, 51
remittance advice and secondary payer, 51–52
sample ASC X12 Institutional Health Care Claim, 48–50
and the use of loops, 46
working with outside entities, 52
business use and definition, 52–53
Trading Partner Agreement (TPA), 52
audit trails, 69, 73, 98
authorization, 23
compared with consent, 23

biologics, 41
biometrics ID, 68, 93
Blue Cross and Blue Shield, 8
Business Associate (BA), 29, 31, 65, 70, 73

Centers for Medicare and Medicaid Services (CMS), 8, 21, 39, 42, 52, 61, 62, 90, 91
CHAMPVA, 6, 18
check digit, 91
Civilian Health and Medical Program for the Uniformed Services (CHAMPUS), 18
clergy, 25, 96
Clinton, Bill, 4
code sets, 38. *See also* designated code sets
communication protocols, 37
Computer-based Record Institute (CPRI), 93

confidentiality. *See* privacy

consent, 22

    compared with authorization, 23

    implied, 22

    written, 22

Consolidated Omnibus Budget Reconciliation Act (COBRA / 1985), 7

Corporate Master Patient Index, 92

covered entity, 18–19, 23

crossover claims, 51

Current Dental Terminology, Version 4 (*CDT-4*), 41

Current Procedural Terminology-4th Edition (*CPT-4*), 40–41

Current Procedural Terminology-5th Edition (*CPT-5*), 41

de-identified health information, 22

Department of Health and Human Services (DHHS), vii, 5–6, 10, 17, 27, 30, 36, 39, 42, 51, 59–61, 71–72, 88–89, 91–92, 94; Office of HIPAA Standards, 71

designated code sets, 39. *See also* ASC X12 standards

    dental, 41

    diagnosis, 39–40

    drug, 41

    inpatient, 40

    non-medical, 42

    outpatient, 40–41

    designated record set, 23

disenrollment, 45

documentation, 95

drugs

    over the counter (OTC), 41

    prescription, 41

electronic data interchange (EDI), 5, 37, 38, 39, 42

electronic signatures, 68–69; and nonrepudiation, 68–69

Employee Retirement Security Act (ERISA / 1974), 6

Employer Identification Number (EIN), 9, 11, 89–90

encryption technology, 70, 73

family members, and patient information, 95

faxing of health information, 98

fraud, 6

Government Printing Office, 21

group health plan, 7

health care clearinghouse, 8, 18–19, 70

Health Industry Number (HIN), 90

Healthcare Common Procedure Coding System (HCPCS), 39, 40–41, 53

    Level II codes, 41

    Level III codes, 41

Health Care Financing Administration, 39

health care provider, 5, 8–11, 18

    and sharing of patient information, 96

    small providers, 11, 71, 90

health identifiers. *See* unique health identifiers

Health Industry Number (HIN), 90

health insurance claims, submission of, 8

Health Insurance Portability and Accountability Act (HIPAA / 1996), vii—viii, 4–5, 11, 17, 51–52, 53, 88–90. *See also* designated code sets; Health Insurance and Portability Accountability Act, titles of; Privacy Ruling; Security Ruling; Transaction and Code Set Ruling; unique health identifiers

    business challenges of, 8–11

    development of, 5–6

    government websites providing information on, 21

    importance of, 94

    myths and misconceptions about, 94–98

    overview, 5

    standardized electronic format of claims, 8

Health Insurance Portability and Accountability Act, titles of, 4, 6

    Title I: Health Care Access, Portability, and Renewal, 6

    Title II: Preventing Health Care Fraud and Abuse, 6–7, 9, 17–18, 20–21

    Title III: Tax-related Provisions, 7

    Title IV: Group Health Plan Requirements, 7

    Title V: Revenue Offsets, 7

    Title XI: General Provisions, 7

    Title XXVII: Assuring Portability, 8

Health Level Seven (HL7), 5

health plan, 18

HIPAA Officer, 19–20, 31, 52, 61

Hobson, David, 5

hospital patient lists, 96

Indian health service programs, 18

Individual Retirement Account (IRA), 7

individually identifiable health information (IIHI), 9, 22, 25, 31, 60
information system, 64
infrastructure, 67
Institutional Review Board (IRB), 26
interactive videoconferencing consultation, 71–72
International Classification of Diseases, 9th Edition, Clinical Modification (ICD-9-CM), 39, 40, 53
International Classification of Diseases-10th Revision Procedure Coding System (ICD-10-PCS), 40
International Revenue Service (IRS), 9, 89
International Standards Organization (ISO), 91

limited data set, 27
long-term care insurer, 18

marketing, 27–28
Mayo Clinic, 93
Medicaid, 6, 41, 90
medical records, 96
Medical Records Institute, 93
Medical Savings Account (MSA), 7, 11
Medicare, 6, 8, 51, 90
Medicare+Choice, 18
Medicare Prescription Drug, Improvement, and Modernization Act (2003), 39
minimum necessary, 20, 28–29, 31, 45, 63, 73, 95
Mitre Corporation, 93
Modifications to Electronic Data Transaction Standards and Code Sets, 36

National Association of Boards of Pharmacy (NABP), 90
National Center for Health Statistics, 39
National Drug Code (NDC) System, 41
National Provider Identifier (NPI), 90, 91
National Uniform Billing Committee (NUBC), 89, 91
National Uniform Claim Committee (NUCC), 89
   Data Subcommittee, 42
need to know, 20
non-medical code sets, 62
   Claim Adjustment Reason Codes, 42
   Claim Status Category Codes, 42
   Claim Status Codes, 42
   Reject Reason Codes, 42
   Remittance Advice Remark Codes, 42
Notice Of Privacy Practices (NOPP), 23, 29–30, 95

Office of Civil Rights (OCR), 18, 21, 30, 96
orthotic devices, 41

passwords, 63, 68, 69
penalties, 30–31, 97
personal identifiers, 22, 91–94
personal representative, 24, 25
policy handbooks, 17–18, 30
preexisting condition exclusions, 6
prescription pickups, 95
press, the, 97–98
privacy, 10, 17–18
Privacy Officer, 20, 30
Privacy Ruling, 9–10, 11, 17, 26, 27, 28, 31–32, 63, 73
prosthetic devices, 41
protected health information (PHI), 20, 62. *See also* Privacy Ruling; protected health information (PHI), and disclosures; Security Ruling
   and Business Associates, 29
   definition of, 21–22
   enforcement guidelines, 30–31
   integrity of, 69
   and radiology film, 22
   use of, 22
   and workforce training, 29–30
protected health information (PHI), and disclosures, 22, 23, 96
   limiting disclosure, 28
   permitted use and disclosure with authorization, 27
      for marketing purposes, 27–28
      and psychotherapy notes, 27
   permitted use and disclosure without authorization, 24
      incidental, 25–26
      for individual access, 24
      when permission is obtained, 24–25
      for the public interest or benefit, 26
      for research, 27
      for treatment, payment, and health care operations, 24
      required, 24
Provider Taxonomy Code, 42

psychotherapy notes, 21
  disclosure of, 27
  process notes, 27
Public Health Act, 6

risk, 61–62
  and adverse threats, 62
risk analysis, 62–63, 73
risk management, 62, 73

Security Officer, 20, 61, 62–63, 67–68, 70–71, 73
Security Ruling, 10–11, 59, 73. *See also* Security
  Officer
  administrative safeguards, 61
    Business Associate contracts, 65
    contingency plan, 64, 73
    evaluation of security, 65
    information access, 63
    security incidents, 64
    security management, 61–62
    security training, 63–64
    workforce security, 63
  challenges to compliance, 72
  core requirements, 59–61
  documentation, 70–71
  excluded items, 60
  impact on organizations, 71–72
  organization requirements, 70
  physical safeguards, 65
    device and media controls, 67
    facility access control, 65–66
    workstation access, 66
    workstation security, 66–67
  technical safeguards, 67–68
    access control, 68–69
    audit controls, 69
    and integrity of PHI, 69
    person or entity authorization, 69
    transmission security, 70
self-insurance, 18

social security number (SSN), 93
Standard Unique Employer Identifier (SUEI),
  89, 90
Standards for Electronic Transactions, 36
  types of, 37–38
subscriber, 45

telemedicine, 71
Trading Partner, 52
Trading Partner Agreement (TPA), 52, 53
Transaction and Code Set(s) Ruling, 10, 11, 89
  purpose of, 37–38
treatment, payment, and operations (TPO), 22,
  24, 30, 31
TRICARE, 6
unique health identifiers, 88, 98–99
  employer identifier, 89–90
  health care provider identifier, 90–91
  health plan identifier, 91
  personal identifiers, 91
    directory service, 93
    biometric, 93
    patient identification system, 93
    personal immutable properties, 93
    public key-private key cryptography
      method, 93–94
    social security number (SSN), 93
  reasons for, 88–89
Unique Patient Identifier (UPI), 93
Unique Physician Identification Number
  (UPIN), 90
Universal Health Identifier (UHID), 92
user, 63

Washington Publishing Company (WPC), 43
Workgroup for Electronic Data Interchange
  (WEDI), 89, 91
workstations, 65, 66, 73
  security of, 66–67
World Health Organization (WHO), 39